The Dynamics of Dialogue

The Dynamics of Dialogue

Edited by

Ivana Markovà and Klaus Foppa

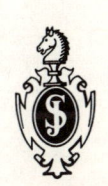

Springer-Verlag New York Berlin Heidelberg
London Paris Tokyo Hong Kong Barcelona

First published 1990

This edition 1990 published by Springer-Verlag New York, Inc.,
175 Fifth Avenue, New York, NY 10010, USA

© Authors and Editors 1990

All rights reserved. This work may not be translated or
copied in whole or in part without the written permission
of the publisher (Springer-Verlag New York, Inc., 175
Fifth Avenue, New York, NY 10010, USA), except for
brief excerpts in connection with reviews or scholarly
analysis. Use in connection with any form of information
and retrieval, electronic adaptation, computer software,
or by similar or dissimilar methodology now known or
hereafter developed is forbidden. The use of general
descriptive names, trade names, trademarks, etc., in
this publication, even if the former are not especially
identified, is not to be taken as a sign that such names, as
understood by the Trade Marks and Merchandise Marks
Act, may accordingly be used freely by anyone.

Printed in Great Britain

Library of Congress Cataloging-in-Publication Data

The Dynamics of dialogue / Ivana Marková, Klaus Foppa, editors.
    p. cm.
    Includes index.
    1. Dialogue. 2. Oral communication. I. Marková. Ivana.
II. Foppa, Klaus, 1930–
P95.455.D96   1991
306.4′4—dc20

Contents

Preface — vii

Introduction *Ivana Marková* — 1

Part I: The foundations of the dialogical approach — 23

1. The social psychology of the prefix 'inter-':
   A prologue to the study of dialogue *Rob Farr* — 25

2. Social communication, dialogue and
   conversation *Thomas Luckmann* — 45

3. Dialogue and dialogism in a socio-cultural
   approach to mind *James V. Wertsch* — 62

4. On axiomatic features of a dialogical approach
   to language and mind *Ragnar Rommetveit* — 83

5. Perspectival structure and dynamics in
   dialogues *Carl F. Graumann* — 105

Part II: Specific aspects of dialogical dynamics — 127

6. A three-step process as a unit of analysis in
   dialogue *Ivana Marková* — 129

7. The power of dialogue dynamics *Per Linell* — 147

8. Topic progression and intention *Klaus Foppa* — 178

vi *Contents*

9. On the local sensitivity of conversation
   Jörg R. Bergmann   201

Name index   227

Subject index   232

Preface

We first met in December 1985 at a seminar on 'The social construction of meaning' held at the Werner Reimers Foundation in Bad Homburg, Germany. We had both been invited by Carl Graumann, and we both presented papers dealing with the dynamic aspects of speech and conversation. During the seminar we realized that we shared many concerns about the study of language, and we decided to establish a study group to explore the dynamic characteristics of speech and conversation. The study group, to be called 'The Dynamics of Dialogue', was to be interdisciplinary, including scholars in the social and human sciences. It would focus on both conceptual and methodological issues. The Werner Reimers Foundation accepted our proposals for this project and agreed to host the study group and invite other scholars to our seminars and conferences.

The group is made up of the following people:

Professor Jörg Bergmann, Department of Sociology, University of Konstanz, Germany;

Professor Rob Farr, Department of Social Psychology, The London School of Economics and Political Science, London, England;

Professor Klaus Foppa, Department of Psychology, University of Berne, Switzerland;

Professor Carl Graumann, Department of Psychology, University of Heidelberg, Germany;

Professor Per Linell, Department of Communication Studies, University of Linköping, Sweden;

Professor Thomas Luckmann, Department of Sociology, University of Konstanz, Germany;

Profesor Ivana Markovà, Department of Psychology, University of Stirling, Scotland;

Professor Ragnar Rommetveit, Department of Psychology, University of Oslo, Norway.

We are extremely grateful to the Werner Reimers Foundation for enabling us to carry out our project. We believe that there are very few places in the world today where scholars from the social and human sciences can meet in such a relaxed atmosphere and hospitable environment to discuss scientific and human issues.

This volume, *The Dynamics of Dialogue*, is the first in a proposed series of the same title. The contributors are the members of the study group, together with Professor James V. Wertsch, Department of Psychology, Clark University, USA, who was invited to contribute a chapter.

We would like to express our gratitude to a number of people. First, to the Werner Reimers Foundation and its director, Mr von Krosigk, for their continuous interest and help. Second, to Mrs Söntgen, who organizes and reorganizes our meetings with the utmost efficiency and who always makes us feel very welcome. Mr Colin Wright of the University of Exeter has given generous help in correcting our English, with editorial work and preparing the index. We are also very grateful to Harvester Wheatsheaf for their undertaking to publish the series, and to Farrell Burnett for her help in the preparation of the book for publication.

Klaus Foppa
Ivana Markovà

Introduction
Ivana Markovà

Why the dynamics of dialogue?

For many readers 'dialogue', i.e. face-to-face interaction between two or more persons using a system of signs, is transparently dynamic. As a dialogue progresses, the participants exchanging both words and gestures, it unfolds, assumes new forms and, finally, terminates. In this sense dialogue is, almost by definition, dynamic. The term 'dynamics' in the title of this book, however, has a much broader connotation than this. Dialogues, like any other kind of social interaction, are always embedded in particular socio-historical contexts that are themselves highly dynamic, be they cultures, institutions or the relationships of power that obtain between the participants. These dynamic contexts are, perforce, also part of the study of dialogue.

In this volume we aim to provide the basis of an appropriate conceptual framework for the study of dialogue as it is embedded in its socio-historical contexts. The authors come from different disciplines within the social and human sciences, and derive their theoretical positions from various traditions including phenomenology, semiotics, pragmatics, the sociology of knowledge, ethnomethodology, symbolic interactionism and German expressivism. As a result, the views expressed in this volume are diverse. Over and above this diversity, however, the authors all share certain fundamental philosophical and epistemological presuppositions, which contribute to the coherence of the volume as a whole. These shared presuppositions are described below.

The interactionist perspective

The authors of this volume all subscribe to what, in today's terms, might be called an *interactionist* perspective. They assume that there is an interdependence between the *agent* and his or her *sociohistorical environment*. These two elements are seen as inextricably interlinked; neither can be defined independently of the other. The assumption of the mutual nature of this relationship between person and environment is a pervasive feature of most phenomenological approaches. Phenomenological analyses focus on individuals' intentional perspective-taking within the contexts of their experience (Graumann, 1988). Over half a century ago, the reciprocity of perspectives between self and other, defined by Schutz (1932) as intentional 'other-orientation', became the basis of his perspectival social theory of knowledge.

The interdependence between individual and environment was also taken for granted by such pragmatists as Dewey and Mead. According to the pragmatists' conception, the relationship between organism and environment is not a one-sided affair, with the organism adapting to its environment and the environment remaining unchanged. Rather, as Mead (1934, pp. 130 and 245–6) made clear, the organism is active in selecting its environment and responding to it in its own unique way, using it purposefully to support its own life-processes. In order to understand the life-processes of an organism, therefore, we must consider the mutual interrelations between organism and environment. Mind, too, is a function of the interrelations between individual and environment.

> Mind . . . lies in a field of conduct between a specific individual and the environment, in which the individual is able, through the generalised attitude he assumes, to make use of the symbolic gestures, i.e. terms, which are significant to all including himself. (Mead, 1922, p. 163)

In his essay 'The objective reality of perspectives', Mead (1927) insisted that conditions only constitute an environment insofar as they affect actual individuals and these individuals only. Human agents are not imprisoned within their own perspectives, but are orientated towards others and the perspectives of those others.

The German expressivists, too, focused their attention on mutual perspective-taking between people. Herder (1877–1913) maintained that in order to understand other cultures and traditions, one must empathize with them, i.e. orientate oneself towards them and examine them on their own, rather than on one's own, premises. It is only through language and self-consciousness that one genuinely directs oneself outward towards others. For Hegel (1807), the mutual relationship between an individual and his or her environment was an indispensable prerequisite for the acquisition of knowledge and the development of self-consciousness. The Russian and Prague semioticians of the 1920s and 1930s (e.g. Vygotsky, 1962; Vološinov, 1973; Mukařovský, 1936, 1976), following the Hegelian line of thought, adopted the viewpoint that all individual actions are social and historical phenomena. For them, just as for Baldwin (1897) and Mead (1934), the individual becomes self-aware in the process of becoming aware of others. Correspondingly, the meaning of words and utterances is always co-determined by speaker and hearer, who both actively enter into the communicative process.

The centrality of symbolic social communication

The second area to unite the authors of this volume is a common belief in the *symbolic nature of human communication* as being central to the study not only of language and speech but also of human social phenomena in general. It is through social communication that the human mind has developed, and that personal, interpersonal, intergroup and intercultural problems are defined and solved, and activities negotiated, normalized and changed. As Luckmann (1984) argues, people do not speak to each other in order to maintain language in being, but in order to do things to each other, with each other, against each other or by themselves. Through social communication people define and construct their social reality, shape it and act upon it; that is why 'languages are at the core of social stocks of knowledge' (Luckmann, *ibid.*, p. 14). It is for these reasons, too, that symbolic social communication is not just a subject to be treated in a single chapter in a textbook of either sociology or social psychology. It is a subject that pervades *all* human social activities, and so it constitutes the very core of social science itself.

What is dialogue?

In the history of studies concerned with language and speech, the terms 'dialogue' and 'dialogical' have been given two fundamentally different yet complementary meanings. Firstly they have been used, in a very broad sense, with reference to a particular epistemological point of view that we shall here call *dialogism* (see also Holquist,

1981). Secondly they have been used, in a much more narrow sense, with reference to symbolic communication that is face to face. In this section I shall discuss both these conceptions, together with their counterparts, monologue and monologism.

Dialogism

Dialogism is an epistemological approach to the study of mind and language as historical and cultural phenomena. The origin of this approach can be traced to the German expressivism of the eighteenth and nineteenth centuries, although the German expressivists did not actually use the term 'dialogism' to identify their point of view. For scholars such as Herder (1771) and Humboldt (1836–9), language and speech were social activities that continue to develop and change. According to this tradition, language and speech originate and develop *through* social interaction and communication. Social interaction and communication, therefore, are absolutely essential to the existence of language and speech as living phenomena; without them, language would remain a relic of our past.

Russian scholars of the early part of this century, such as Bakhtin (1981) and Vološinov (1973), valued very highly the contribution made by the German expressivists to the study of language and speech, and built on this tradition in their own work. 'Dialogue', Vološinov maintained, 'can be understood in a broader sense, meaning not only direct, face-to-face, vocalized verbal communication between persons, but also verbal communication of any type whatsoever' (Vološinov, 1973, p. 95). For example, a verbal performance in printed form, such as a book, is also a form of verbal communication, and understanding it is a dialogical enterprise. The writer or poet aims to reach his or her potential readers by imagining how they might respond to his or her work, whilst readers, for their part, actively search for the writer's or poet's intended meanings (Rommetveit, 1974). Analysing the prose of the Czech writer and dramatist Karel Čapek, Mukařovský (1939/1964), a distinguished Prague semiotician, emphasized that the essence of Čapek's writing is to carry on a conversation with his reader.

> The reader here is a silent partner in the conversation, who is constantly being told that his opinion of the matter is important; to him are addressed the minute, humorous distortions of reality, on his emotional participation are calculated the lyrical passages; here we can really begin to speak of an *interpenetration of prose with dialogue*. (*ibid.*, p. 147, emphasis added)

The dialogism of George Herbert Mead (1934) is clearly expressed in his view that social interaction is an evolutionary and sociohistorical process that has led to the development of symbolic communication and to the appearance of mind. 'Mind arises through communication by a conversation of gestures in a social process or context of experience – not communication through mind' (Mead, 1934, p. 50).

In all these conceptions of dialogism it is presupposed that the knowledge of language and communication can be advanced only by the study of speech in concrete societal and historical contexts.

Monologism

Dialogism as an epistemology contrasts sharply with monologism. Monologism takes as its starting point language as a ready-made, normative and static system of signs. Thus Humboldt (1836–9) argued that just as an anatomist dissects a dead body into its parts in order to examine its structure, so a philologist dissects language into single monological utterances, and examines them closely by themselves, as abstractions. The spectre of the philologist dissecting language in a monological fashion as if it were a dead body has been a recurrent concern of social psychologists of language throughout the history of the study of language. Vološinov (1973) complains that philologists commonly start their investigations with a finished monological utterance, which he describes as 'the ancient written monument'. He maintains that an ostensibly monological utterance is an abstraction and that an utterance can be studied, meaningfully, only as an inseparable element of verbal communication. Every utterance is a link in a chain of speech actions and its meaning can be discovered only by studying it in relation to the speaker's intentions. A supposedly monological utterance is really an *active* response of the speaker to something that preceded it, and it is calculated, in return, to produce an *active* response. In contrast to this view, Vološinov continues, the philologist is concerned not with an active, but with a completely passive kind of understanding. Being preoccupied with the study of dead languages only, the philologist takes an 'isolated monument', i.e. a single utterance, and relates it to other such monuments rather than to its use in a real flow of human communication.

Mead (1934), in similar vein, argued against the philologist's approach to the study of language. He maintained that the philologist, when studying language, often takes as his or her starting point the situation of a prisoner in a cell. The prisoner knows that other prisoners are in a similar position to his or her own, being shut up in neighbouring cells, and so attempts to establish some arbitrary method of communication, such as tapping on the wall. The point of this example is that the philologist, in order to study language, presupposes individual consciousness and then asks how the language of the individual can become a social affair.

This criticism of individualism and of the static perspective in language must not be taken as a rejection of philology and linguistics as disciplines. Relatively static and individual perspectives in language have just as important roles to play as the dynamic and social ones. However, the static and individual perspectives must be studied *together with* the social and dynamic perspectives in a dialogical relationship. This point of view was already being clearly expressed early this century by semioticians such as Vygotsky, Vološinov, Mukařovský and Karcevskij. Several authors in this volume argue very strongly that the study of mind and language must be based on a dialogical relationship between the individual and social planes of cultural development (see Wertsch, Chapter 3) and between the relatively static and dynamic perspectives of language and mind (see Luckmann, Chapter 2; Rommetveit, Chapter 4; Graumann, Chapter 5; Marková, Chapter 6). Monologism as an epistemology ignores these dialogical relations, and takes as its point of departure only the individual and static aspects of language and mind.

Dialogue

The second of the two conceptions of dialogue enumerated above is a narrow one that restricts dialogue to symbolic face-to-face oral and gestural communication. The special characteristics of dialogue in this narrower sense are a result of interaction, in temporal and spatial *immediacy*, between two or more participants who face each other and who are intentionally conscious of, and orientated towards, each other in an act of communication (Schutz, 1932). However, when interlocutors respond instantly to each other, they respond to far more than just the immediacy of each other's gestures and utterances. Their gestures and utterances convey past experiences and cultural knowledge which may, or may not, be shared. The extent of their common stock of knowledge and their mutual acquaintance with each other is reflected in the kind and quality of the dialogue they hold. For example, Birdwhistell (1970), in his descriptions of shared family codes in communication, refers to the expertness of his mother in 'untalk', commenting that her silences were louder than all his father's machinery. The Russian semiotician Yakubinsky (1923/1986) made the same point in his excellent essay (yet to be translated into English), 'On dialogical speech'. The more the interlocutors share a common experience and the more they are able to assume each other's perspective, the more they can abbreviate their speech and communicate through such incomplete forms of speech as hints, or even through the first letters of words, as Kitty and Levin do in Tolstoy's *Anna Karénina* (1875–7) (Vygotsky, 1962; Yakubinsky, 1923/1986).

These examples make it clear that this form of dialogue is defined as face-to-face symbolic communication *between persons*. Characteristics such as immediate intentional perspective-taking, shared sociocultural experience and mutual knowledge between participants exclude from this definition other kinds of communication that sometimes, metaphorically, are called dialogue, e.g. person–animal and animal–animal communication or person–computer interaction. These kinds of communication, though important in their own right, are not discussed in this book.

The conception of dialogue as face-to-face interaction is of crucial importance for the understanding of language change. This was emphasized by German expressivists such as Humboldt, for whom language develops when humans communicate with one another; 'As a phenomenon . . . language develops in social intercourse and humans understand themselves only by having tested the comprehensibility of their words on others' (Humboldt, 1836–9, p. 36). Through hearing the sound of a word produced by another the meaning of that word is 'objectified', i.e. it becomes part of the social reality. Thus, it is through interindividual communication that concepts and words become public property. The richer and the more varied the forms of social intercourse, the more language profits, because it is 'forged by speaking' (Humboldt, *ibid.*, p. 127).

It is through the mutual exchange of ideas, i.e. through speech, that human beings stimulate each other. The individual's power to think 'is fired by its equivalent' (Humboldt, *ibid.*, p. 36), it requires the presence, either actual or imagined, of someone else. Humboldt explains his claims by saying that if one strives for truth on one's own there is always the danger of self-deception: one must always test one's own ideas against those of other human beings to see where one is going. Social intercourse is one of the most powerful media for verifying one's own ideas. However, Humboldt insisted, 'conversation is never comparable to the transmission of information'. Unfortunately, 150 years later information-processing models of communication and sender–receiver models of language production and understanding still predominate. Graumann (1986, p. 11) sums up the situation.

> The present process of 'cognitivation', i.e. of explaining more and more psychological phenomena in terms of the information-processing paradigm, diminishes rather than improves chances to account for the social context of verbal and nonverbal behaviour.

The essential role of conversation for the intellectual, emotional and artistic development of people was also emphasized by Lazarus (1879). He maintained that a scholarly and scientific study of conversation has been totally neglected, probably because science professes to be concerned with universals and general principles of nature. Since each conversation is manifestly different from all other conversations, science has the problem of bridging the gap between the specific and the general. Lazarus, like Humboldt, argued that conversation is fundamental to the development, maintenance and sharpening of thinking. Individuals engaged in conversation are mutually involved with each other. They test their ideas against each other, take each other's point of view and mutually influence one another as persons. In a science of conversation, Lazarus contended, various issues needed to be studied, including evolutionary aspects of, and the psychological mechanisms involved in, speech, and the classification of different kinds of conversations and their social contexts.

Wundt (1916) argued that language was the product of people. As Farr (1983) has pointed out, the significance of Wundt's folk psychology lies primarily in his emphasis on culture. Wundt turned his attention to the linguistic and expressive analysis of dialogue and to the gesture-language of primitive people and of the 'deaf and dumb'. For him, the origin of human language was to be found in the development of human gesture, particularly in its expressive, imitative and pantomimic functions. Following Wundt's work, Mead (1934) developed his conception of the human gesture. In contrast to Wundt, whose concept of gesture was based on Darwin's study of the expression of emotions, for Mead 'a gesture was a part-action which *others* completed' (Farr, 1980). Mead focused his attention on vocal gesture in dialogue as a form of stimulation that plays a vital role in the development of the self. He pointed out that while we cannot see ourselves when our face assumes a certain expression we can hear the tone of our voice while speaking. We respond to the quality of our voice in the way that others respond to it and in this way we monitor and control it (Farr, this volume, Chapter 1).

Yakubinsky (1923/1986) argued that dialogue as face-to-face interaction is a natural, and genetically primary, form of speech and language. He was concerned with the variety of social functions that speech fulfils. These functions are evident not only in the many languages, dialects and speech types that characterize particular social groups, but also *within* the same language or dialect. Following Humboldt, Yakubinsky drew attention to the many different forms of expressive speech, such as conversation, poetry, prose, rhetoric and science which can coexist within the one language. These forms of expressive speech serve different goals in social communication, and the study of these goals must not be ignored.

Monologue

Yakubinsky (1923/1986) was critical of contemporary linguistics for neglecting the study of different forms of speech expression and their functions. He, himself, concentrated on two basic forms of speech expression: dialogue and monologue. Monologue, as the counterpart to dialogue considered as a form of face-to-face interaction, must be distinguished clearly from the monologism discussed earlier. Monologism is the epistemology of individualism. In contrast, monologue is unequivocally *dialogical* in nature. In dialogue, as has been pointed out above, the participants rely on obtaining *immediate* response from each other, whether verbal or gestural. Monologue, likewise, is directed towards the other person, in the extreme case, that other person being the self. However, it does not rely, or relies only partially, on immediate feedback from the other.

The distinction between dialogue and monologue is often a difficult one to make. For example, although the participant may be in a state of temporal and spatial immediacy with his or her interlocutor, he or she may become totally encapsulated in his or her own point of view whilst engaged in a dialogue with the other. Descriptions of one's own feelings, experiences and points of view, and long passages of speech in which little or no attention is paid to one's interlocutor, are examples of 'monological dialogues' in which the speaker is temporarily orientated more towards an internal conversation with him- or herself rather than towards his or her interlocutor. Foppa (this volume, Chapter 8) discusses the role of such monological dialogues with respect to topical progression in conversation.

At the other end of the continuum is genuine monologue, for

example prose that the writer transforms into a dialogue. An instance of such a case is Čapek's prose mentioned above (see page 4). Mukařovský (1939/1964), in his analysis of Čapek's prose, pointed to the linguistic aspects of this transformation of a monologue into a dialogue. The prose proceeds as if it were a conversation between two persons, yet without quotation marks to separate the utterances of one person from those of the other. In the example from Čapek the dialogue is carried out between the hero of Čapek's novel, Hordubal, and a cowherd. Hordubal, returning from America to his native village, is walking along a slope and looking at himself with the eyes of a cowherd on the opposite slope. He then invents a dialogue between the cowherd and himself, which is purely the product of his imagination. As Mukařovský (1939/1964, p. 149) puts it, in Čapek's writing, prose has finally changed when it has 'absorbed the dialogue into itself'. This change of a monologue into a dialogue actually enriches the style of writing by the use of dialogical devices such as interrogatives, declaratives and exclamatory intonation, achieving a more dramatic and intimate impact on the reader than the writer would have achieved using a prosaic style alone. Contrasting dialogical and monological speech, Foppa (this volume, Chapter 8) makes similar observations. As dialogue and monologue are transient forms of speech, they often cannot easily be categorized as strictly one or the other.

It was Yakubinsky's distinction between dialogue and monologue that Vygotsky took up in his account of inner speech, arguing that inner speech is intrinsically social. For Vygotsky, too, dialogue was the starting point for the study of speech. In child development, speech is originally external to the child in the sense that he or she speaks in order to address others but not him- or herself. Only when speech has become *externally* established, *for others*, can it then also become *internalized*, i.e. *for oneself*. In other words, the child can have a *monologue* with him- or herself only after he or she has developed the ability of holding a *dialogue* with others. Thus, internalized or monological speech in the child is not egocentric in the Piagetian sense, but is social speech that has reached a higher stage, being for self.

It is against the background of these conceptions that the contributors to this volume test and develop their own ideas concerning the dynamics of dialogue. In order to accommodate both uses of the term 'dialogue', we shall distinguish between them consistently in the following way. The noun 'dialogism' will be used with reference to a broad epistemological view of the nature of knowledge with respect to language and mind. The noun 'dialogue' will then refer to dialogue in the narrow sense, that is, to reciprocal face-to-face interaction using symbolic language. The adjective 'dialogical', however, will be used in both the broad and the narrow sense.

Concepts and methods in the dialogue analysis

Throughout the history of the natural and social sciences there have been persistent difficulties with the conceptual and methodological analysis of inherently dynamic phenomena. The reason for this is that, from its very beginnings, the fundamental preconception of Western science has been that truth is uncovered by searching for the underlying, *invariant*, characteristics and laws of both natural and social phenomena. From Plato to Descartes and beyond it has been generally assumed that although such phenomena change in the course of time, their 'essences', whatever that term may mean, must surely be immutable and timeless. Consequently it has been believed that phenomena only really become intelligible when their supposed ultimate invariable characteristics have been discovered. Hierarchically structured tree diagrams of sentences as models of speech production and comprehension (Linell, 1982), and tree diagrams of semantic memory (Markovà, 1982) are examples that testify to such beliefs. Inevitably, scientific concepts and methods of analysis reflect this search for the immutable and timeless characteristics of things and events, treated as independent and discrete entities.

The search for invariants seems to be ubiquitous in human thought. We shall see later in this section, however, that in dialogical epistemology invariants are viewed only as *temporarily* static or frozen perspectives of the *changing* world.

Against Cartesian individualism

Although the problems of dynamic phenomena and change were addressed in Greek philosophy by such philosophers as Heraclitus and Aristotle, it has only been in the last 200 years, with the emergence of the ideas of biological and socio-historical evolution, that the problem of how to conceptualize dynamics and change has been addressed in the natural and social sciences. The epistemology of dialogism that has resulted from these evolutionary ideas has become a serious rival to Platonic–Cartesian monologism, challenging its presupposition of the existence of discrete, immutable and timeless entities. For example, Herder (1771) argued persuasively against the individualistic and rationalistic theories of language set forth by Condillac, Rousseau and Süssmilch. Some 100 years later we find Baldwin (1911) insisting that individualistic theories ignored the social origins of knowledge and should 'be laid away in the attics where old intellectual furniture is stored'. Mead (1934), too, rejected the individualistic assumptions of both the rationalists and the empiricists, who claimed that individual minds are logically prior to the social processes in which they are embedded. The criticisms of monological 'abstract objectivism' by Russian semioticians in the 1920s (Vološinov, 1973; Bakhtin, 1981) are remarkably similar to those made by Mead and Baldwin. More recently, in the 1960s and 1970s, scholars objecting to Chomskyan psycholinguistics (Uhlenbeck, 1973; Rommetveit, 1974) were concerned with the same problems, arguing against the assumptions underlying the study of utterances *in vacuo* and the search for *invariants* in the meanings of words appearing in different contexts.

The basic presuppositions of abstract objectivism, individualistic theories of knowledge, logical atomism and positivism, and Chomskyan psycholinguistics are all rooted in the same Cartesian paradigm (Markovà, 1982). The criticisms of cognitivism in the social sciences in the 1980s still address the same kind of Cartesian presuppositions (Costall and Still, 1987; Linell, 1982, 1988; Winograd and Flores, 1986). Clearly, then, these Cartesian presuppositions have still not been exorcised, but keep reappearing under various aliases and in different guises, in Western philosophical and scientific thought. They are so deep-rooted in our intellectual inheritance that when they enter, stealthily, into our concepts, theories and methods of analysis they thrive concealed, often being promulgated, unwittingly, by those who claim to offer an alternative to Cartesian dualism.

Temporal fixations of perspectives

In order to be generally accepted by the academic world, the epistemology of dialogism has to cope with certain difficulties that are due to cultural biases inherent in Western thought. These are due, as Rommetveit (this volume, Chapter 4) points out, to the fact that the presuppositions on which our study of cognition and communication are based have been only *partially* reflected upon, and therefore our speculations about language and thought have not been based on the true *perspectivity* that is essential to dialogical epistemology. Our inability to acknowledge fully our presuppositions, Rommetveit maintains, stems from the fact that many of them are *universally shared*, due to environmental, biological and social constraints. Precisely because they are universally shared (Rommetveit, *ibid.*, p. 89), these background conditions are inaccessible to our reflective consciousness and so remain 'entirely unacknowledged as long as they stay fixed'. For example, the environment that sustains various human traits and capacities has been relatively stable for up to 100,000 years, a period of time that appears to be sufficient for the traits and capacities themselves to become relatively stable (Schilcher and Tennant, 1984). As genetic information becomes encoded in an organism and is transmitted from generation to generation within an environment stabilized for that purpose, not only does it appear to be no longer affected by the environment, but the organisms' autoregulatory feedback systems buffer out the effects of variations in that environment (Lewontin, 1982, p. 155). Once phenomena become thus stabilized and their knowledge commonly shared, they induce presuppositions of the existence of stabilized and timeless invariants, and confidence and belief in the relatively stable world around us, and so tend to conceal from reflexive consciousness the ubiquitous perspectival relativity of knowledge.

A medical photographer, in capturing dynamic phenomena in the real world, e.g. a diseased part of the body, temporarily freezes the movement in an event. Moreover, in order to obtain different perspectives of the diseased part, the photographer takes pictures from various positions, using different lighting. Yet the doctor, before making a decision with respect to the patient's treatment, must not only take all these photographic perspectives together, he or she must also consider the patient as a whole, the possible prognoses of the disease and other circumstances that might mitigate against or facilitate the healing process. Taking into consideration the global situation of the patient the doctor must start with the assumption that the disease itself is dynamic and that what he or she gets from the photographer's pictures is nothing but *temporal fixations* of dynamic phenomena.

Just as a photographer freezes the movement in an event in a photographic image, so the researcher may mentally freeze phenomena that are dynamic, in order to examine them (see Rommetveit, this volume, Chapter 4). However, it must be understood that such a temporarily fixed image of a dynamic phenomenon serves only a heuristic purpose and must on no account be mistaken for the concept that properly represents the dynamic nature of the phenomenon itself. Once the temporarily stabilized image is conceptualized, it must be tested against the phenomenon it is intended to explain.

Dialogical logic

Dialogism is guided by the principles of logic that have been called *dialogical, dialectical* or *co-genetic*. It is a logic of the interdependence between phenomena and it starts with *wholes* rather than with *parts of wholes*. The difference between wholes and parts is a matter of the kinds of relationships into which they can enter. Logical atoms, as the units of analysis in traditional formal logic, have been assumed to have *external relationships* with other atoms and so to be combinable or divisible into complex aggregates (Russell, 1914; Stebbing, 1933). Wholes, as units in dialogism, cannot be analysed into component parts simply because there are no such parts. Each supposed 'atomic part' exists only in an interdependent relationship with other parts. For example, and as discussed earlier, an organism is defined in terms of the environment to which it belongs; the meaning of a linguistic item can be defined only in terms of the speaker who utters it and listener towards whom it is directed; and so on. The wholes, so defined, are bound by *internal relations* rather than by external relations, and dialogical (dialectical, co-genetic) logic is defined as the study of such relations.

The basis of co-genetic logic as the logic of systems in development was laid down by Hegel (1812–16). Similar ideas concerning co-genetic logic have emerged recently (see Spencer-Brown, 1969; Barwise and Perry, 1983; Rommetveit, this volume, Chapter 4). The prefix 'co-' in 'co-genetic logic' expresses the point of view that both the supposed 'atomic part', and its counterpart with which it forms the whole, co-develop mutually through their progressive interdependent differentiation and transformation. Co-genetic logic is concerned with language change and with intentionality (see Foppa, this volume, Chapter 8).

If one adopts co-genetic logic as a guiding principle for the study of such a dynamic phenomenon as a *dialogue*, then the challenge is to state precisely what the *units* of analysis of dialogue are. Whatever these units may be, they must coexist in a dynamic relation to each other. For example, if perspectival relativity is an essential feature of dialogue, it must also be implicit in the units of analysis used. If a dialogue forms an ecologically inseparable whole with its socio-historical context, the units of analysis chosen must also imply this relationship (Markovà, this volume, Chapter 6). Moreover, linguistic items fulfil different functions not only in different communicative contexts but also within one particular communicative context. They are involved in mutual dependencies with the speakers and their social environment at several different levels at the same time. The units of analysis of dialogue must cope both with such multilevel dependencies and with the different messages that interlocutors deliver. However, in order to analyse the dynamics of dialogue, it may be necessary, as with certain concepts, to treat the units of analysis, temporarily, as if they were stable.

The elaboration of dialogical concepts and the task of establishing the most appropriate units of analysis of dialogue form an ambitious programme for the future. In its discussion of the issues outlined above, this volume is intended as a significant contribution towards such a programme.

The contents of the book

This book, which is the first volume of a proposed series, *The Dynamics of Dialogue*, focuses primarily on fundamental conceptual and epistemological problems, and on historical issues in so far as they relate to current concerns in the study of mind and language. In addition, some of the authors also address more specific questions of method and analysis of the dynamics of dialogue.

The first part of the volume, 'The foundations of the dialogical approach', starts with Farr's contribution, which focuses on the centrality of communication in the human and social sciences and on the meaning of dialogicity in terms of the *interrelationship* between individuals, groups and their social environment. Farr views these interrelationships as already grounded in phylogenetic and ontogenetic, as well as in historical and cultural phenomena. Thus, he refers in various places to 'the social psychology of the prefix *inter-*' found in such terms as inter-action, inter-personal, inter-relational, inter-view, and argues that this usage is an explicit marker of inherently social forms of psychology and of psychological forms of sociology. It is a fundamental presupposition in the work of Wundt, Tarde, Mead and Ichheiser, and in the work of more recent scholars such as Goffman, Heider, Jones, Davis and Nisbett. Social psychology that fails to conceptualize interrelationships between phenomena and that does not acknowledge their centrality in the study of mind and behaviour falls necessarily into the traps of individualism. It is because of his emphasis on the centrality of the prefix *inter-* that Farr calls his chapter 'A prologue to the study of dialogue'.

Farr emphasizes that speech must be studied as both action and reflection of mind. Although this claim may not appear, at first sight, to need any justification, Farr shows how difficult it is to conceptualize the inter-relationship between mind and behaviour in a truly dialogical manner. Social scientists have, for a long time, been preoccupied with the question as to which comes first: mind or behaviour. Farr argues that contemporary cognitive science, focusing one-sidedly on the study of mental processes only and failing to acknowledge the action-based nature of language, has been unable to grasp the dialogical inter-relationship between mind and action (or behaviour). In contrast, this inter-relationship was conceptualized in a dialogical manner by Mead and the semioticians of the early part of this century, and it is also taken for granted in phenomenologically orientated theories of knowledge.

Taking a broad evolutionary perspective of dialogicity, Luckmann in Chapter 2 is concerned with the differences between the concepts 'social communication', 'dialogue' and 'conversation'. Reminding the reader that more complex forms of symbolic interaction have their roots in non-symbolic social communication, he identifies the most important dimensions of social communication, namely sociality, reciprocity, abstraction and intentionality. These dimensions are combined in different ways in the communication of various animal species. Such combinations display diverse qualities, forms and levels of flexibility from one animal species to another.

Human languages differ from other systems of social communications in a fundamental way: they not only result from biological evolution but also from socio-historical and cultural development. Dialogue has evolved from complex chains of communicative human actions through an entangled combination of conscious, subconscious, intentional and automatic responses, some of which are phylogenetically very old while others are relatively young. Luckmann argues that although it may be impossible to disentangle all these complexities, one should be aware of their existence within different layers of human communication. Dialogue seems to be a universal form of human communication, although some of its important characteristics are limited to certain historical and cultural periods. For example, equality in the participants' communicative status is not a universal characteristic of dialogue and occurs only in *conversation*, a historical subspecies of dialogue. The importance of Luckmann's contribution lies not only in his conceptual analysis of social communication and its semiotic forms, but also in his emphasis of the central role of communication in the human and social sciences.

The theme concerned with the meaning of the prefix inter- introduced by Farr, reappears in Wertsch's contribution (Chapter 3). Discussing Vygotsky's *genetic method*, Wertsch warns about a possible misinterpretation of the meaning of the transition from inter- into intra-individual psychological processes. According to Vygotsky, the child's cultural development proceeds on two planes: on the social, i.e. *interpsychological* plane, and on the individual, i.e. *intrapsychological* plane. The transition from the former to the latter plane is known as *internalization*. Wertsch points out, however, that internalization does not simply mean that the individual's mental activity grows out of social experience. Rather, mental activity proceeds on both planes at the same time, reshaping structures and functions in them both. Thus, the relationship between inter- and intra- is itself a genetic process in which the structure and function of mental activity in both planes changes through developmental transitions between them.

Wertsch makes the important claim that one does not need to be concerned with comparative studies between cultures and societies in order to pursue socio-cultural analyses of mind. Instead, one can examine social communication and mental processes as embedded in cultural, historical and institutional settings. Developing his own ideas of a socio-cultural approach to mind and language, Wertsch pays particular attention to the work of Vygotsky and Bakhtin.

The Bakhtinian theme of *voice* is elaborated by Rommetveit in Chapter 4. Rommetveit argues for co-genetic logic, which he sets against formal logic, in the study of mind and language, and for perspectival relativity approaches to knowledge. He maintains that mainstream cognitive science, which is based on the assumption of Cartesian monologism, does not see its method of exploration and its concepts as in any way temporary. Rather, it treats them as being entirely objective and as having universal validity. In assuming that it has emancipated itself from human values and motives and that it presents a pure and neutral scientific point of view, cognitivism deceives itself: 'what appears as *emancipation* from human concerns from within the enclaves of scientific enquiry is from a dialogical and co-genetic point of view, *fixation*' (Rommetveit, this volume, p. 94). From the dialogical standpoint, any neutrality and purity of scientific facts that is devoid of perspective-taking is purely fictitious. Perspectivity is always present where human consciousness is involved and must be allowed for in all scientific thinking.

Graumann's chapter is concerned with the perspectival structure of dialogue. He introduces the topic of dialogical perspectivity by a discussion of two complementary aspects of dialogue: the conceptualizations of *what* is going on in a dialogue and of *who* is participating in a dialogue. He characterizes perspectivity as the common structure of cognitive experience between the interlocutors, and pinpoints intentional reference as its basic constituent. Graumann draws on phenomenological literature and on the work of

Schutz, Mead and Litt who developed the conception of perspectival structure in cognitive experience. The structure of reference not only establishes cognitive space, it also involves a dynamics of its own which, in social interaction, presupposes perspective-setting and perspective-taking. Graumann raises the question of how the basic mutuality of perspective-taking shows itself in a dialogue. He discusses the triple reference in discourse, i.e. topic, hearer and self, in establishing a common cognitive space, and gives special attention to the mutually perspectival evolution of topics. Thus to Graumann, dialogicity means primarily perspective-setting, perspective-taking and multiperspectivity of cognition.

The second part of the volume, *Specific aspects of dialogical dynamics*, starts with Markovà's chapter which in a way bridges the concerns of the two parts. In addition to conceptual issues, Markovà raises the question of what kind of units of analysis would cope with the dynamic nature of dialogue. She argues that the units of analysis of dialogue must be based on a co-genetic logic involving three steps. This is so because each dialogical unit is itself a dynamic process and as such must maintain the characteristics of the dynamics of dialogue. These include the mutuality between the individual and his or her social environment, temporality, internal relations and foregrounding. Three-step units of analysis can be identified at different levels of the analysis of dialogue, such as at the level of word, utterance, turn or any more inclusive speech action.

Although dialogue is always embedded in its social, cultural and historical contexts, it must also be viewed as a sequence of interlocking utterances in which speakers take each other's perspectives, set their own perspectives, negotiate their positions and attempt to dominate each other. In fact, as Luckmann maintains in Chapter 2, while dialogue is defined as reciprocal symbolic interaction, most dialogues are *asymmetrical* in the sense that participants, in one way or other, express, or attempt to express, their dominance and power over each other. In Chapter 7, Linell makes an important contribution to these areas. He shows that asymmetries can be studied at different levels, starting with the one that is most local from an utterance-to-utterance point of view, and finishing with the one defined by the speakers' roles within different social contexts and institutional frameworks. He distinguishes between several kinds of dialogical dominance and focuses on the study of *interactional dominance*. Linell explores certain characteristics of interactional dominance using his initiative–response method of analysis. The method concurs with the basic idea of co-genetic or dialogical logic according to which each unit of analysis is defined in terms of three steps. In Linell's method, each unit of analysis is a *result* of both an *initiative* that introduces something new into an interaction, and a *response* to some previous speech events. While initiatives and responses can be documented at a microlevel of utterance-to-utterance, they also form aggregated patterns over sequences of utterances, and these patterns may characterize dialogues of certain kinds.

Many dialogical interactions can be analysed in terms of three-step models in which both participants take their turns and mutually work towards their communicative goal. Foppa, however (Chapter 8), raises a question about interactions in which one interlocutor has a predetermined communicative aim and ignores the intentions and goals of his or her interlocutor. In this case, the dynamics of a dialogue are determined primarily by the firm intentions of one of the participants, namely, the one who violates the rules of mutual turn-taking. Although dialogues of this kind are fairly common, there has been little attempt by psycholinguists and by social psychologists of language to explore the role of *intention* in communication. Foppa draws the distinction between the type of dialogues in which interlocutors speak without a particular intention and those that are guided by strategic intentions. Topic progression in dialogue may occur in both of these types. Foppa points to the difficulties of identifying intentions in dialogues and to conceptual problems involved in the definition of intention. Like Mukařovský, Foppa claims that there are no fundamental differences between monologue and dialogue, although a dialogue offers a greater variability of topics and the topic progression is more dynamic than in a monologue. Focusing on intention and topic progression, Foppa opens up an intriguing and largely unexplored territory of theoretical and methodological interest.

The issue of topic development is also taken up by Bergmann in his chapter on the local sensitivity of conversation. A conversation is usually characterized by progression and maintenance of a topic jointly produced and coherently formulated by the speakers. Yet the speakers are also sensitive to local, i.e. situational, matters that are not part of the conversational exchange. Local sensitivity means openness towards environmental matters that can be exploited for conversational purposes of one kind or another. For example, local objects may suddenly attract the speakers' attention and become topicalized. Topicalization of such objects can be an important device for starting a conversation with strangers, avoiding silences when conversation is slowing down, or averting communicational disharmony. However, only some types of discourse allow topicalization of situational matters. In other cases, specifically those of institutional discourse, which have predefined goals, topicalization would be destructive or even offensive, and local sensitivity has to be kept under strict control. In the dynamics of dialogue, speakers' local sensitivity is a highly functional means of achieving perspectivity and enhancing dialogicity in the flow of talk.

The authors of this volume are aware that many of the issues they raise remain, at present, unresolved at both the theoretical and the methodological levels. They have sought to offer here merely the basis of an epistemology of dialogism, leaving room for various themes to be taken further in their future work. Such an approach is justifiable by the very method they advocate. Dialogism is about the development of ideas in the science of human mind and language. It is through 'dialogue' that the authors propose to advance our knowledge of language and mind.

References

Bakhtin, M. M. (1981), *The Dialogic Imagination: Four essays by M. M. Bakhtin*, M. Holqist (ed.), trans. C. Emerson and M. Holquist, Austin: University of Texas Press.

Baldwin, J. M. (1897), *Social and Ethical Interpretations in Mental Development*, London: Macmillan.

Baldwin, J. M. (1911), *The Individual and Society*, London: Rebman.

Barwise, J. and Perry, J. (1983), *Situations and Attitudes*, Cambridge, Mass.: MIT Press.

Birdwhistell, R. L. (1970), *Kinesics and Context*, Philadelphia: University of Pennsylvania Press.

Costall, A. and Still, A. (eds) (1987), *Cognitive Psychology in Question*, Chichester and New York: Wiley.

Farr, R. M. (1980), 'Homo loquens in social psychological perspective', in H. Giles, W. P. Robinson and P. M. Smith (eds), *Language: Social psychological perspectives*, Oxford and New York: Pergamon.

Farr, R. M. (1983), 'Wilhelm Wundt (1832–1920) and the origins of psychology as an experimental and social science', *British Journal of Social Psychology*, 22, 4, 289–301.

Graumann, C. F. (1986), 'Language – the interface between individual and social', *Newsletter of the Social Psychology Section of the British Psychological Society*, 15, 5–19.

Graumann, C. F. (1988), 'Phenomenological analysis and experimental method in psychology – the problem of their compatibility', *Journal for the Theory of Social Behaviour*, 18, 33–50.

Hegel, G. W. F. (1807), *The Phenomenology of Mind*, trans. J. B. Baillie (1949), London: George Allen & Unwin; New York: Macmillan.

Hegel, G. W. F. (1812–16), *Science of Logic*, trans. A. V. Miller, London and New York: George Allen & Unwin, 1969; New York: Humanities Press, 1976.

Herder, J. G. (1771), 'On the origin of language', in *Sämtliche Werke*, B. Suphon (ed.), reprinted, Hildesheim: Georg Olms, 1967.

Herder, J. G. (1877–1913), *Sämtliche Werke*, B. Suphon (ed.), reprinted, Hildesheim: Georg Olms, 1967.
Holquist, M. (1981), 'The politics of representation', in S. Greenblatt (ed.), *Allegory in Representation: Selected papers from the English Institute*, 163–83, Baltimore: Johns Hopkins University Press.
Humboldt, W. von (1836–9), *Über die Kawi-Sprache auf der Insel Java*, I–III, Berlin: Königliche Akademie der Wissenschaften.
Lazarus, M. (1879), 'Über Gespräche', in M. Lazarus *Ideale Fragen in Reden und Vorträgen*, Berlin: Hofmann.
Lewontin, R. C. (1982), 'Organism and environment', in H. C. Plotkin (ed.), *Learning, Development and Culture*, Chichester: Wiley.
Linell, P. (1982), *The Written Language Bias in Linguistics*, Studies in Communication, 2, Linköping: University of Linköping Press.
Linell, P. (1988), 'The impact of literacy on the conception of language: the case of linguistics', in R. Saljo (ed.), *The Written World*, Berlin and New York: Springer.
Luckmann, T. (1984), 'Language in society', *International Social Science Journal*, 36, 5–20.
Markovà, I. (1982), *Paradigms, Thought and Language*, New York and Chichester: Wiley.
Mead, G. H. (1922), 'A behaviourist account of the significant symbol', *The Journal of Philosophy*, 19, 157–63.
Mead, G. H. (1927), 'The objective reality of perspectives', in E. S. Brightman (ed.), *Proceedings of the Sixth International Congress of Philosophy*, New York: Longmans, Greens and Co., 1927. Reprinted in A. J. Reck (ed.), *Released Writings, George Herbert Mead*, Chicago and London: The University of Chicago Press, 1964.
Mead, G. H. (1934), *Mind, Self and Society*, Chicago: Chicago University Press.
Mukařovský, J. (1936/1976), 'L'art comme fait sémiologique', in E. Rádl and Z. Smetáček (eds), *Actes du Huitème Congrès International de Philosophie à Prague 1934*, Prague: Organizační Komitét Kongresu. Trans. as 'Art as semiotic fact', in L. Matejka and I. R. Titunik (eds), *Semiotics of Art*, Cambridge, Mass.: MIT Press, 1976.
Mukařovský, J. (1939/1964), 'Próza Karla Čapka jako lyrická melodie a dialog', *Slovo a Slovesnost*, 5, 1–12. Trans. as 'K. Čapek's prose as lyrical melody and as dialogue', in P. L. Garvin (ed.) *A Prague School Reader on Esthetics, Literary Structure and Style*, Washington, DC: Georgetown University Press, 1964.
Rommetveit, R. (1974), *On Message Structure*, New York and London: Wiley.
Russell, B. (1914), *Our Knowledge of the External World*, London: George Allen & Unwin.
Schilcher, F. von and Tennant, N. (1984), *Philosophy, Evolution and Human Nature*, London: Routledge & Kegan Paul.
Schutz, A. (1932), *Der Sinnhafte Aufbau der Sozialen Welt. Eine Einleitung in die verstehende Soziologie*, trans. as *The Phenomenology of the Social World*, Evanston, Ill.: Northwestern University Press, 1967.
Spencer-Brown, L. (1969), *Laws of Form*, London: George Allen & Unwin.
Stebbing, S. (1933), 'Logical positivism and analysis', *Proceedings of the British Academy*.
Tolstóy, L. (1857–77), *Anna Karénina*, 3 vols, Moscow, 1878.
Uhlenbeck, E. M. (1973), 'Semantic representation and word meaning', in E.

M. Uhlenbeck, *Critical Comments on Transformational-Generative Grammar*, 1962–72, 135–57, The Hague: Smits.

Vološinov, V. N. (1973), *Marxism and the Philosophy of Language*, trans. L. Matejka and I. R. Titunik, New York and London: Seminar Press.

Vygotsky, L. S. (1962), *Thought and Language*, New York: Wiley.

Winograd, T. and Flores, C. F. (1986), *Understanding Computers and Cognition: A new foundation for design*, Norwood: Ablex Publications.

Wundt, W. (1916), *Elements of Folk Psychology*, trans. E. L. Schaub, London: George Allen & Unwin; and New York: Macmillan.

Yakubinsky, L. P. (1923/1986), 'O dialogiceskoi reci', in L. P. Yakubinsky, *Izbrannye Raboty*; reprinted in A. A. Leotjev (ed.), *Yazyk i ego funkcionirovanije*, Moscow: Nauka.

PART I
The foundations of the dialogical approach

1 | The social psychology of the prefix 'inter': A prologue to the study of dialogue

Rob Farr

Department of Social Psychology, The London School of Economics and Political Science

The dynamics of a three-person group is dramatically different from that of a two-person group. This is so because it is possible to form coalitions in the former size of group, but not in the latter. Those who study the dynamics of small groups claim that an increase in size from two to three is qualitatively different from any further increase in size beyond three (Simmel, 1955a,b; Caplow, 1968; Cartwright and Zander, 1954). I am perfectly happy to accept that this is so. I wish merely to add that the study of the dyad differs, often dramatically, from the study of the individual. The difference can amount to a difference between two rival paradigms for research – the Hegelian and the Cartesian (Markovà, 1982). The interactions *between* individuals are generally of greater significance than the actions of individuals. The latter, indeed, are only understandable in the context of the former, and it is probably artificial to distinguish between the two – although one can say that the former are genetically prior to the latter. I would argue that what is happening between individuals is more significant than what might be happening within the mind of any one individual. The difference between interactions and actions is contained in the prefix 'inter'. This is what I mean by the social psychology of the prefix 'inter'. When, *inter alia*, we consider language, dialogue is a prologue to monologue. It can only be considered appropriately, I shall argue, within a Hegelian, rather than within a Cartesian framework.

Rival epistemologies

Mead's critique of Wundt's philosophy of mind

Psychology, as an experimental science, was conceived, broadly, within a Cartesian framework. Whilst Wundt was not, strictly speaking, a Cartesian, he did not have an explicitly social model of mind when he established psychology as the science of mental life (Farr, 1987). His experimental science depended largely, though not exclusively, on the use of introspection. The events that formed the basis of the oral report occurred in the mind of the person whom we would now identify as the subject of the experiment. The objects of study in Wundt's ten-volume *Völkerpsychologie* (1900–20), on the other hand, were language, religion, customs, myth, magic and related phenomena. These are collective mental phenomena. They are the products of the interactions of the many. There was, clearly, a contrast between his experimental study of consciousness and his collective psychology. The difference, in part, is one of levels. Wundt, however, lacked the theoretical and conceptual tools that would have enabled him to inter-relate these two forms of psychology. The requisite theoretical conceptions were worked out by G. H. Mead (1934), who had studied with Wundt at Leipzig. In his social philosophy Mead demonstrated how 'self' emerges out of social interaction. In the course of evolution humans became 'minded organisms'. This is the phylogenetic context for the emergence of self. The self then emerges, ontogenetically, in the development of individual members of the species. Mead worked backwards from Wundt's *Völkerpsychologie* and, in so doing, he developed an explicitly social model of mind (Farr, 1987). Mead showed how mind and self are social emergents 'and that language, in the form of the vocal gesture, provides the mechanism for their emergence' (Morris, p. xiv, in Mead, 1934).

It was the Cartesian dualism implicit in Wundt's conception of consciousness that Mead found unacceptable. Mead directly challenged Wundt's assumption that consciousness is a uniquely individual phenomenon: he showed how a person's self-awareness (i.e. his or her awareness of him- or herself as an object in the social world of others) arises from interacting with those others in the course of growing up. In this way he demonstrated the purely social antecedents of individual consciousness. As a major pragmatist philosopher, Mead set himself the task of refuting the Cartesian dualism of mind and body which had bedevilled the birth of psychology as an experimental discipline. His arguments against Cartesian dualism were based on a close reading of Darwin. In Mead's thought, mind and self are intimately interlinked. 'The body is not a self, as such; it becomes a self only when it has developed a mind within the context of social experience' (Mead, 1934, p. 50). Mead interpolated the notion of 'self' between the model of 'mind' that underlay Wundt's experimental science and the model of 'society' that underlay his *Völkerpsychologie*. This accounts for the logical progression of Mead's course of lectures in social psychology, i.e. mind, self and society (Mead, 1934).

Wundt's treatment of language and Mead's elaboration thereof

In the writings of Wundt there are at least three treatments of language that are distinguishably different. The first concerns his intuitive insight, based on his reading of Darwin, that the origins of language are probably to be found in gesture. This is worked out in the opening chapters of the first volume of his *Völkerpsychologie*, in which he describes the sign languages of deaf mutes, American Indians, Cistercian monks and Neapolitans. Mead started the development of his social psychology, at Chicago, from Wundt's concept of 'the human gesture' (Mead, 1934). This is why Mead is probably correctly classified as a 'social behaviourist', i.e. the notion of gesture is central to the whole of his social psychology. (It is no accident, I would claim, that C. W. Morris, the editor of Mead's lectures in social psychology, went on, in *Foundations of the Theory of Signs* (Morris, 1938) and *Signs, Language and Behavior* (Morris, 1946), to establish semiotics on a purely behavioural basis.)

Mead, on reading the opening volumes of Wundt's *Völkerpsychologie*, immediately appreciated the significance of Wundt's proposal that the origins of language are to be found in gesture (Mead, 1904). He correctly perceived that Wundt was claiming language to be the special province of the psychologist. Mead's brilliant elaboration of Wundt's idea is central to my presentation in this chapter. Mead's treatment of language is much more dialogical than Wundt's. The evolutionary antecedents of the use, by humans, of language as a means of communication are to be found in the 'conversation of gestures' that characterizes a fight between two dogs or two cats or between a dog and a cat such as Darwin described in *The Expression of the Emotions in Man and Animals* (Darwin, 1872). Mead went on to show how language results from a complication in the system of gestures that is peculiar to the human species. He treats language in the context of social interaction. The prefix 'inter-' (as in, for example, symbolic *inter*action) is integral to Mead's elaboration of Wundt's ideas.

For Mead, Darwin provided the necessary antidote to a purely Cartesian treatment of language. Language was no longer an ethereal or disembodied phenomenon. Wundt, in his concept of the 'human gesture', provided Mead with the clue he needed to solve the problem. Luckmann (this volume, Chapter 2) takes up this aspect of language in his discussion of dialogue in face-to-face interaction.

A second aspect of Wundt's treatment of language relates to the fact that he did not entirely escape the Cartesian dualism that had also infected his experimental science. This is clearest when he talks about the psychology of the sentence. For Wundt, the sentence was the most characteristic unit of human language. This is why Blumenthal (1975) is able to claim, with some justice, that Wundt is the founding father of modern psycholinguistics. Modern psycholinguistics, however, is shot through with Cartesian assumptions. These assumptions are quite explicit in the case of Chomsky. The Cartesian assumptions underlying modern psycholinguistics have been criticized, from a social psychological perspective, by Rommetveit (1968, 1974, 1984) and Marková (1982). According to Blumenthal, for Wundt 'sentences can be studied from the point of view of how they express a thought or from the point of view of their physical shape. The problem of the transformation from the inner to the outer state was thus a key issue for him' (Blumenthal, 1973, p. 12). Sentences, however, are disembodied utterances. Wundt's discussion of the psychology of the sentence is even compatible with the jargon of the modern telecommunication engineer, with its talk about the 'encoding' and 'decoding' of messages.

Mead, of course, rejected this aspect of Wundt's treatment of language – largely for the reasons outlined above. For Wundt, language was the product of mind; for Mead, mind was the product of language. There is a dramatic difference between these two positions. As Wundt's theory of language *presupposed* the existence of mind, the latter was left as something mysterious and unexplained (rather like Descartes' ghostly conception of the mind). Mead was much bolder and more radical in his thinking than Wundt. He showed how mind emerges 'naturally' out of the 'conversation of gestures', and how this occurred, phylogenetically, in the emergence of the species, and occurs again, ontogenetically, in the development of each individual. 'Mind arises through communication by a conversation of gestures in a social process or context of experience – not communication through mind' (Mead, 1934, p. 50). Elsewhere, I have commented:

> It was Köhler, I believe, who said that 'it is easier, starting with behaviour to include mind than it is starting with mind to include behaviour'. Wundt, attempting the latter of these two tasks, was forced to separate his social psychology (based on language conceived as a form of gesture) from his mental science (based mainly, though not exclusively, on the use of introspection). Mead, in the light of Wundt's experience, was able to *reverse* this process – starting the development of his social psychology from Wundt's concept of the gesture he then went on to explain the inherently social nature of mind i.e. starting with *behaviour* he *was* able to include mind. In his social psychology mind became a natural phenomenon and so ceased to be mysterious. (Farr, 1987, p. 9)

The third distinct aspect of Wundt's treatment of language was his belief that language was an important component of culture. In this respect Wundt was an important influence on both Boas and Sapir. The origins of this tradition are to be found in the work of the German expressivists – Humboldt, Herder and Hegel (Marková, 1983). This German tradition of research, regarding language as a social phenomenon, was also important in the evolution of Soviet psychology (see Wertsch, this volume, Chapter 3). For Wundt it was impossible to study higher cognitive functions in humans within the laboratory by means of introspection.

> It is true that the attempt has frequently been made to investigate the complex functions of thought on the basis of mere introspection. These attempts, however, have always been unsuccessful. Individual consciousness is wholly incapable of giving us a history of human thought, for it is conditioned by an earlier history concerning which it cannot of itself give us any knowledge. (Wundt, 1916, p. 3)

It is this aspect of language that Luckmann (this volume, Chapter 2) refers to as a socio-historical a priori.

If Wundt's experimental science was Cartesian, his *Völkerpsychologie* was more Hegelian in its inspiration. By juxtaposing the collective with the merely individual, Wundt created the antithesis that Mead was later to resolve as he developed his own form of social psychology.

The Cartesian paradigm in the historical development of psychology

Descartes' philosophy was inimical to the development of the social sciences. His method of radical doubt had led him to doubt whether other people had 'minds', but had left him in no doubt that he, himself, had one. As a result we have both a mental philosophy of the 'self' and a behavioural science of the 'other' (Meyer, 1921). When psychology first became an experimental science it was the science of mind and it depended largely on the use of introspection. This was not a particularly viable form of science. When observer and observed are one and the same person, as occurs in the case of introspection, it is impossible to obtain an independent check on the veracity of the observations that serve as the basis of such a new science. Science is a public enterprise and it cannot be based on such private data. This was why Mead was critical of the philosophy of mind that underlay Wundt's experimental science.

In the history of psychology, narrowly conceived as an experimental science, behaviourism is usually presented as the antidote to the failings of 'mentalism'. Indeed behaviourism was a crusade to rid psychology of the notion of mind. Psychology rapidly ceased to be the science of mind and became, instead, the science of behaviour. It was thought, falsely as it transpired, that behaviourism had finally laid to rest the ghost of Descartes. The mental philosophy of self had been banished and the behavioural science of the other had been enthroned. This, however, was still Cartesianism. Marková (1982) has observed that the history of Western philosophy is often presented as a conflict between 'rationalism' and 'empiricism'. This, in her opinion, obscures the fact that they are actually both part of the Cartesian paradigm. The real incommensurability between rival paradigms, according to Marková, is between Descartes and Hegel. I would similarly want to argue that the apparent antithesis, in the history of experimental psychology, between 'mentalism' and 'behaviourism' obscures the fact that they both belong to the same Cartesian paradigm. Not only did Descartes create a dualism between mind and body; he also created a dualism between self and other. It is this latter dualism that has proved inimical to the development of the social sciences. 'Philosophical concentration on the problem of the relation of the mind to the body reduced the study of society to the problem of whether other minds existed' (Friedman, 1967, p. 163). The prefix inter- helps to couple that which Descartes cut asunder.

The Hegelian and pragmatist alternatives

It is the interrelationship between self and other that is the true antidote to Cartesian dualism. This is to be found in the phenomenology of Hegel and in the pragmatism of G. H. Mead and C. S. Peirce. In his attack on the Cartesian theory of knowledge, Peirce argued that the knowledge which each of us has of him- or herself as a unique thinking subject is not as obviously intuitive as Descartes had supposed it to be.

> A plausible conclusion . . . is that our self-knowledge is always in fact inferential, although the inferences on which it is based have become for the most part so habitual to us, and as a result of this habituation so 'telescoped', that we very easily come to regard our self-knowledge as immediate or intuitive. (Gallie, 1952, p.66)

The self for Mead is not a disembodied self. I am an object in the social world of other people and as a result of *inter*acting with those others I become an object to myself. The action, so to speak, is in the interaction – hence the importance of the prefix inter-. Dialogue and conversation are important expressions of that process. Language plays a crucial role for Peirce, as well as for Mead:

> while . . . we never succeed in 'seeing ourselves' *exactly* 'as others see us', or in seeing others exactly as they see themselves; nevertheless we do – if Peirce's view is correct – see ourselves, as others do, through our speech and the rest of our interpretable behaviour; and we see others (as they see themselves) through *their* speech and other interpretable behaviour. The important consequence is, that our knowledge of our own thoughts, and hence the possibility of our controlling, developing, and criticising them, is not essentially different from our knowledge of, and hence our power to influence, the thoughts of others. In other words, whenever we think we are in effect communicating – seeking to persuade or instruct or perhaps simply questioning – either covertly with ourselves or overtly with other people. 'All thinking', Peirce writes, 'is dialogic in form. Your self of one instant appeals to your deeper self for his assent'. (Gallie, 1952, p. 82)

Much of the psycholinguistic tradition of research in modern psychology is Cartesian in its inspiration. The controversy between Chomsky and Skinner, for example, over the former's review of the latter's *Verbal Behavior* (Skinner, 1957), is really a linguistic equivalent of the debate between rationalists and empiricists in Western philosophy. As has been noted above, both of these philosophical traditions are part of the Cartesian inheritance.

The either/or and the both/and phases in the development of psychological science

The social psychology of mind and behaviour

To date, in the course of its short history, psychology has been *either* the science of the mind *or* the science of behaviour. It has never been both at one and the same time. Nor has it ever really succeeded at being either, because first of all mind, and then behaviour, were conceived of in non-social terms. What is needed now is a social psychology of *both* mind *and* behaviour. The current preoccupation with cognitive science is but a half-way house on the road back to psychology becoming, once again, the science of mental life (Farr, 1987). Wundt created *both* an experimental science *and* a social psychology, but he was unable to move freely between the two. A difference of level was involved, such as that between the individual and the collective, and while Wundt's experimental science was non-social, his social psychology was non-experimental. By adopting the social behaviourism of G. H. Mead I am endeavouring to develop an experimental social psychology that is concerned with *both* mind *and* behaviour (Farr, 1978).

The key to developing such a psychology is to be found in the social psychology of the prefix inter- as it appears in such compound words as *inter*-actions, *inter*-faces, *inter*-views and *inter*-personal relations. Cognitive science lacks, as yet, an adequate theory of consciousness. It would be all too typical if, when it did acquire one, it ceased to be the science of cognition and it had become, once again, the science of mind (Farr, 1987). I have indicated above reasons (mainly those of Rommetveit and Marková) for believing that the conception of language that informs modern cognitive science is Cartesian in its inspiration. In the sense in which Marková (1982) uses the word paradigm, there has not yet been a shift in paradigm in the historical development of experimental psychology. She uses the term to refer to the Cartesian and Hegelian paradigms in the history of Western philosophy. The shift from the science of mind to the science of behaviour is still within the Cartesian paradigm. So, too, is the shift from behavioural science to cognitive science. To escape from the impasse of Cartesian dualism, it is necessary to adopt either a Hegelian or a pragmatist paradigm. Psychology might have to cease being a branch of the natural sciences and become, instead, an explicitly social science.

Adoption of the social psychology of the prefix inter- would enable us to move out of the either/or phase and into a both/and phase in the development of psychological science. By judicious use of this prefix in theoretical formulations we could overcome the dualities *within* experimental psychology *and* move *between* different levels of explanation in the social sciences. This, in turn, would enable us to overcome such false antitheses as those between mind and behaviour or between self and other, *and* to link up consciousness, mind or cognition with society or culture through the agency of self and the medium of language.

The social psychology of the inter-view

In Farr (1984) I sketched the outline of a social psychology of the inter-view. There, I defined an inter-view as 'a technique or method for establishing or discovering that there are perspectives or viewpoints on events other than those of the person initiating the interview' (*ibid.*, p. 182). There is an explicit recognition in this approach that more than one perspective is involved when two or more persons interact. It is an approach that recognizes the inter-face that lies at the heart of the inter-view. I accept the arguments of Becker and Geer (1957) for the superiority of participant observation as a method of research over an exclusive reliance upon the interview *per se*. The advantage of participant observation is that it retains, within the one methodology, the divergent perspectives of both the actor and the observer. By the simple expedient of adding a hyphen, i.e. by writing about inter-views rather than interviews, I have sought to make the inter-view equivalent to participant observation and to highlight its inherently social nature. It is important, in my opinion, to remind observers (particularly those who are psychologists) that they are also participants, and to remind participants that they are also observers. What is novel about this approach to inter-viewing is the salience of the prefix inter-.

I have approached the dynamics of the inter-view from the differing perspectives of both the actor and the observer (Jones and Nisbett, 1972). One fails to grasp the significance of what is happening in the course of an inter-view if, in the interests of science, one's attention is focused exclusively on what can be observed directly from the outside. This limited perspective came into psychological science with the acceptance of behaviourism. As early as 1896, Dewey had warned of the dangers of accepting the reflex arc as the basic unit of behaviour. He and Mead were academic colleagues at the time, and his article was based on extensive discussions between the two men. Why, Dewey argued, should one focus on that segment of the act that is visible from the perspective of an outside observer? The beginning of an act is not visible from the outside but first forms in the mind of the actor. Mead went on to elaborate a whole philosophy of the act, in which the perspective of the actor is quite different from that of the observer. In psychological research the dominant perspective has been that of the observer. In connection with the social psychology of encounters, Goffman (1956) has done much to make salient the perspective of the actor. I have drawn heavily on Goffman's work in my outline of the social psychology of the inter-view.

The divergence in perspective between actors and observers

It is important, first of all, to recognize that there is indeed a divergence in perspective between actors and observers. Given this divergence, it is important not to privilege, in the interests of science, one or other of these two perspectives. In the Leipzig laboratory in Wundt's day it was the perspective of the actor (or reagent) that was dominant, i.e. the person who provided the introspective report. Yet at that time observer and observed were one and the same person. With the advent of behaviourism it was the perspective of the observer that became dominant. Observer and observed were now usually two different entities or persons. The reality, if not the theory, was social. When the *Gestalt* psychologists migrated from Germany to America they reintroduced into American psychology the perspective of the actor and they became, in this respect, important forerunners of the cognitive revolution that began to gather momentum in the mid- to late 1950s. These various transitions are part of the either/or phase in the development of psychological science. It is time, now, to move on to the both/and phase of development. It is important, however, to understand just how the two perspectives interrelate. The persons best qualified to solve this particular problem, in my view, are social psychologists.

My account, thus far, of the historical progression of psychological science is seriously misleading. It suggests a simple alternation between the perspectives of the actor and of the observer. The reality is otherwise. The prevailing perspective is that of the observer, even though behaviourism is no longer the dominant force it once was in psychology. I believe this is so because leading psychologists continue to think of their discipline as a branch of the natural sciences. Watson sought to make it so by declaring it to be the science of behaviour. In the natural sciences, vision is the dominant modality of investigation. Forms of psychology based on listening rather than on observing, e.g. psychoanalysis, are accorded a low status in terms of their scientific merits. Whilst behaviourists observe, psychoanalysts listen. Social psychologists who elicit self-reports from their informants are judged, by their more positivist cousins, to be dealing with 'soft' data. Behavioural evidence, i.e. the 'facts', is visible and can be agreed between observers. This constitutes 'hard' data. The preference in scientific circles within psychology for vision over hearing did not cease with the demise of behaviourism as the dominant paradigm for research.

According to Jones and Nisbett (1972), there is a pervasive tendency for actors to believe that their actions are appropriate to the circumstances in which they find themselves, whilst observers of those same actions tend to attribute them to the stable, dispositional characteristics of the actors. This is why Jones and Nisbett refer to a *divergence* in perspective between actors and observers. This divergence, I have argued elsewhere (Farr and Anderson, 1983), is in the visual modality. As our eyes are at the front of our heads we are only rarely objects in our own visual field. This is why there is a divergence in perspective between actors and observers. As a species we are not so self-reflexive in the visual modality as we are in the auditory modality. Tony Anderson and I have argued (*ibid.*) that the divergence in perspective between speaker and listener is not as sharp as that between actor and observer. It is, in fact, more of a convergence than a divergence. This is because we hear ourselves speak more or less as others hear us. This observation is an integral part of the social psychology of G. H. Mead. The convergence in perspective between speaker and listener also explains why radio is a more intimate medium of broadcasting than television. The close link between speaking and listening is crucial, also, to an understanding of the dynamics of dialogue.

The convergence in perspective between speaker and listener and the dynamics of dialogue

More attention needs to be given by psychologists to language and speech if they are to contribute, usefully, to our understanding of the dynamics of dialogue. At present social psychologists understand the visual better than they do the auditory aspects of social encounters. This is why the present chapter is subtitled 'A prologue to the study of dialogue', rather than being concerned with the study of dialogue *per se*. Conversation analysts focus primarily on auditory aspects of dialogue, often neglecting the importance of the purely visual aspects of such social encounters. Clearly we need a both/and approach to the study of dialogue rather than this either/or approach. Conversation analysts sometimes deliberately restrict the conditions under which they elicit their samples of spontaneous conversation in order to minimize or tightly control the visual aspects of the interaction. They do so by, for example, analysing only telephone communications, or using computer-controlled maze games as the principal topic of reference in the conversation between isolated individuals (Anderson and Garrod, 1987; Garrod and Anderson, 1987). These approaches are only minimally social. The theories advocated in the present volume are much more explicitly social in their nature.

The perspective of the actor has never been a particularly salient one in purely psychological traditions of research. The Wundt model of experimental psychology was a comparatively short-lived one and even here the actor was more passive than active (he was sometimes referred to as the re-agent). The cognitive model within American social psychology, introduced by the *Gestalt* psychologists, was only one of a variety of different traditions within cognitive science. In several of the others, the model of cognition is not even a human one. In information technology, for example, the language is that of the telecommunications engineer; in artificial intelligence it is that of the computer scientist. It will be clear from the rest of this chapter that, in developing the perspective of the actor, I have had to borrow most of my models from sociological traditions of social psychology, such as the social behaviourism of G. H. Mead, Goffman's work on the presentation of self in everyday life and Ichheiser's sociology of interpersonal relations.

I have argued that vision is the dominant modality of investigation in psychological science. If psychologists are to contribute, significantly, to our understanding of the dynamics of dialogue then they have to be concerned not only with vision, but also with hearing. They have to be concerned not only with the divergence in perspective between actor and observer, but also with the convergence in perspective between speaker and listener. Most of the literature in experimental social psychology treats actors and observers as different persons, so that a given person is either the one or the other. Clearly each of us is both an actor and an observer. A model capable of capturing this feature is the social and reflexive model of man to be found in the writings of G. H. Mead (Farr, 1987). More recently Bem (1967), who is very much a minority figure in experimental social psychology, has proposed a theory of self-perception where speaker and listener can be either two separate persons or one and the same person. His model is entirely consistent with that of G. H. Mead, though I shall not be examining it further in this chapter.

The sociology and the psychology of interpersonal relations

Newcomb's study of communicative acts

Newcomb used the prefix inter- as a marker in developing his own brand of social psychology. His classic textbook, *Social Psychology* (1952), bore the subtitle, in the revised edition, 'A study of human interaction' (Newcomb, Turner and Converse, 1965). Newcomb believed that the study of social interaction set social psychology apart from all other forms of psychology. He was the architect of a programme of social psychology, at the University of Michigan, that was common to both psychology and sociology. His insistence on the importance of 'communicative acts', as in his classic study of 'the acquaintance process' (Newcomb, 1961), led to his theoretically significant notion of 'strain toward symmetry' in small social networks. This was an important counterweight to the many purely cognitive models of consistency within the minds of individuals that so preoccupied experimental social psychologists at the time. Newcomb (1968) stressed inter- rather than intra-personal balance.

Heider's psychology of inter-personal relations

The whole aim of Heider's project was to create a psychology of interpersonal relations (Heider, 1958). He found that the conception of the psychological life-space of the individual, developed by his friend Lewin (1935), was insufficiently social to serve his own purpose of constructing a psychology of inter-personal relations. There was no way, within Lewin's system, whereby the life-space of one individual could be represented, psychologically, within the life-space of another individual. The key phenomena for Heider, as for Newcomb, were of an inter-actional nature, though Newcomb was much more explicit than Heider with regard to the *social* nature of these interactions. The prefix inter- was important to Heider in that it enabled him to establish a link between the psychological world of one individual and the behaviour of others. Heider highlights the inter-face between self and other, between mind and behaviour. The face at the inter-face between self and other is one's own face.

Heider was centrally concerned with self/other relationships. Hence the importance for him of the prefix inter-. His social psychology is dialectical in nature. It is more Hegelian than Cartesian in its inspiration. In Heider's nomenclature O stands for Other. This is a purely relational term. It makes sense only in relation to the Self. P, i.e. the Perceiver, therefore, stands for Self. In my opinion Heider was insufficiently explicit about this in his psychology of inter-personal relations. P represents the Perceiver's perspective on the world, provided he or she is awake and has his or her eyes open. Remember, however, that P, considered from the perspective of O as a P, is an O. He or she becomes an Other to him- or herself by virtue of being an Other to Others. Hence the awareness of self as an object, which is Mead's definition of self-consciousness. Heider does not just present a psychology of 'the Other One' (Meyer, 1921). That would be behaviourism. That would be part of a Cartesian paradigm. He presents, instead, a social psychology of Self in relation to the Other One, and this is something quite different. It is more Hegelian than Cartesian. The difference between these two paradigms is conveyed by the use of the prefix inter-.

There is an important difference, likewise, between gaze and mutual gaze (see Argyle and Cook, 1976). It is the latter that makes one self-conscious. Ichheiser (1949) was aware of the importance of mutual gaze to the dynamics of inter-personal relations. 'Looking at each other is the most primary form of conversation' (Ichheiser, 1949). It is the origin of our awareness both of others and of ourselves (Marková, 1987). Heider was a strongly visual theorizer, but he was more concerned with gaze than with mutual gaze. He did not elaborate greatly on the various states of awareness of others and of self to which his theory of inter-personal relations gave rise. Mead developed a much more explicit theory of the human self. This, I believe, is because he had a far better appreciation than Heider of the evolutionary significance of language (Farr, 1987). Heider's treatment of language is rather restricted. This may be, in part, because a significant portion of his professional life in America was spent, together with his wife Grace, working with the deaf. His treatment of language, in his classic text *The Psychology of Interpersonal Relations* (Heider, 1958), was more in the tradition of analytic philosophy than in the study of language as a mode of communication. He was concerned, for example, to explicate the meanings of such words as 'can', 'tries', 'ought', etc. In the development of his theoretical ideas, he has been much more directly concerned with vision than he has with either speech or hearing.

Ichheiser's sociology of inter-personal relations

In 1949, Ichheiser published a monograph on *Misunderstandings in Human Relations: A study in false social perception* in which he sought to identify, in the field of social cognition, analogues of the visual illusions that are studied by experimental psychologists. These are common sources of misunderstanding occurring in the relationships that humans establish one with another. As all relationships between humans are also inter-relationships, the prefix inter- is central to Ichheiser's concerns. His monograph was a plea for the importance of studying 'impressions'. The impressions that form in the minds of others have important social consequences for the persons of whom they are impressions. They have the full ontological significance of a Durkheimian 'social fact'.

Ichheiser's monograph was intended as a contribution to the series of monographs on the sociology of knowledge that Mannheim was then editing, in London, at both the London School of Economics and the Institute of Education. It was also a contribution to the study of the ideology of success and failure as this had developed within certain Western cultures in the course of the nineteenth century and into the twentieth. The centre-piece of this ideology is a collective representation of the individual as someone who is responsible for his or her own actions in life. This collective representation is often incorporated within the legal codes of the cultures in which it obtains: individuals who are found guilty of committing criminal acts are punished unless it can be argued, by invoking the McNaughton rules for example, that this particular individual was not responsible for his or her own actions.

It is on the basis of this same collective representation that we praise people when they succeed in life and blame them when they fail (Farr and Moscovici, 1984). Heider (1958) drew on the work of Ichheiser, a fellow Austrian, when elaborating his ideas about the typical attributions that we make concerning the successes and failures both of others and of ourselves. The broader cultural factors identified by Ichheiser are important in the context of the dynamics of dialogue. But social encounters occur within a wider cultural context, and it is important to know this wider context if one is to understand the dynamics of what transpires in the course of any ongoing social interaction.

There is also a much more specific sense in which the work of Ichheiser is relevant to an understanding of the dynamics of dialogue. In the course of his monograph (1949), Ichheiser stated that it is important to distinguish between 'expression' and 'impression'. He argued that Darwin (1872) was not always clear about the nature of this distinction in his book *The Expression of the Emotions in Man and Animals* though he did not elaborate on why he believed that Darwin was confused on this particular issue. Darwin described the impressions that form in the mind of an observer when confronted by the expressive behaviours of a whole range of other species, including the human species. Mead had been critical of Darwin for suggesting that the *purpose* of these behaviours was the expression of the emotions. For Mead speech was a form of expressive behaviour that created more or less the same impressions in the mind of the speaker as it did in the minds of other listeners. Many non-verbal forms of communication, however, create impressions in the minds of observers that are quite different from those that the actor intends. Impressions can have a life of their own that is quite independent of the person of whom they are an impression. This is the point of Ichheiser's monograph. It is a plea for the importance of studying these impressions. He intended his monograph as a contribution to the sociology of knowledge. It became, instead, a contribution to the information-processing paradigm within the study of social cognition, i.e. its social significance was rapidly lost.

The social psychology of encounters and the presentation of self in everyday life

I believe that Erving Goffman successfully identified most of the major components that are important to an understanding of the social psychology of encounters. He focused mainly on the visual aspects of such encounters, i.e. on the divergence in perspective between actor and observer. A performance is an event that is both enacted, by actors, and witnessed, by observers. Goffman was also interested in the analysis of dialogue – his doctoral thesis concerned the use of language in an island community (the Shetland Islands off the north coast of Scotland). However, it was only in his final book (Goffman, 1981) that he took up the topic of dialogue again. In this chapter I shall use the work of Goffman in order to identify the limited and partial insights that social psychologists can provide for understanding the dynamics of dialogue. My strategy is very similar to that of Becker and Geer (1957), who chose to describe the all-inclusive methodology of participant observation in order to highlight the limitations of the interview *per se*. The study of inter-actions is crucial to the whole corpus of Goffman's writings. His studies of dialogue, whilst being more limited in their scope, need also to be set in this wider, more inclusive, context. His social psychology lies broadly within the Meadian tradition of social psychology at the University of Chicago, and he was specifically influenced by the social psychology of Gustav Ichheiser.

Goffman (1956) picked up Ichheiser's suggestion concerning the value of distinguishing between expression and impression and came up with a theory of the expressive behaviour of actors in the social scene that takes into account the impressions forming in the minds of the audience for whom the performance is being staged. Goffman recognized that impressions are 'given off' (i.e. inadvertently) as well as 'managed'. He sought to restore a measure of control to the actor in the social scene. Ichheiser had accorded impressions the status of being social facts in the full Durkheimian sense of the term. Goffman showed how they might be managed – thus restoring some degree of autonomy to the actor. Goffman was centrally concerned with the presentation of self in everyday life. The self is the self that one is in the eyes of others. It refers to one's various situated identities. Whilst researchers may be participant observers *of* the social scene, actors are observing participants *within* it. They are capable of monitoring the impressions they create.

The twin masks of tragedy and comedy which adorn theatres or appear as emblems on theatre programmes symbolize the inter-face between actor and audience. Actors and audiences are on two different sides of these masks. The voice of the actor sounds *through* (*per sonare*) the mask and the audience forms its own impression of the personality of the character being portrayed on the stage. In the theatre, as in everyday life, props provide important cues concerning the personality of their owners – the word personalty, in English, is an old legal term meaning all one's worldly goods. Ichheiser gave an account of the impressions that formed in his own mind concerning the personality of a famous writer he was about to meet, based on the furniture in the author's apartment and the expressive characteristics of the handwritten letter of invitation. He showed how serious mismatches can occur between appearances and reality. His 1949 monograph carries the subtitle 'A study in false social perception'.

We seem to have lost, in non-social forms of psychology, the 'social reputation' approach to the study of personality. At least it is preserved within such sociological traditions of social psychology as those of Ichheiser and Goffman. Psychologists have focused too exclusively on accounting for expressive behaviour and have failed to study, simultaneously, the impressions that form in the minds of others on the basis of that expressive behaviour. It is probably more accurate to say that psychologists, themselves, have become the victims of what Ross (1977) terms 'the fundamental attributional error', this being that instead of treating traits or attitudes or other dispositional entities as *inferences* in their own minds, psychologists have treated them as characteristics of the central nervous systems of the persons they observe. Ross derived his fundamental attributional error from Jones and Davis (1965) and Jones and Nisbett (1972) who, in their turn, derived it from Ichheiser (1949). And so we come back, full circle, to a sociological form of social psychology. The use of the prefix inter- will act as a timely reminder of the need to study the inter-relationship between expression and impression. This may hold in check the operation of the fundamental attributional error.

References

Anderson, A. and Garrod, S. C. (1987) 'The dynamics of referential meaning in spontaneous conversation: Some preliminary studies', in R. G. Reilly (ed.), *Communication Failure in Dialogue and Discourse*, Amsterdam: North Holland.
Argyle, M. and Cook, M. (1976), *Gaze and Mutual Gaze*, Cambridge: Cambridge University Press.
Becker, H. S. and Geer, B. (1957), 'Participant observation and interviewing: A comparison', *Human Organisation*, 16, 28–32.
Bem, D. (1967), 'Self perception: An alternative interpretation of cognitive dissonance phenomena', *Psychological Review*, 74, 183–200.
Blumenthal, A. L. (1973), Introduction to W. Wundt, *The Language of Gestures*, The Hague: Mouton.
Blumenthal, A. L. (1975), 'A re-appraisal of Wilhelm Wundt', *American Psychologist*, November, 1081–8.
Caplow, T. (1968), *Two Against One: Coalition in triads*, Englewood Cliffs, N.J.: Prentice Hall.
Cartwright, D. and Zander, A. (1954), *Group Dynamics: Research and theory*, London: Tavistock Publications.
Darwin, D. (1872), *The Expression of the Emotions in Man and Animals*, London: Appleton.
Dewey, J. (1896), 'The reflex arc concept in psychology', *Psychological Review*, 3, 357–70.
Farr, R. M. (1978) 'On the social significance of artefacts in experimenting', *British Journal of Social and Clinical Psychology*, 17 (4), 299–306.
Farr, R.M. (1984), 'Interviewing: An introduction to the social psychology of the inter-view', in C. L. Cooper and P. Makin (eds), *Psychology for Managers* (second edition), London: Macmillan.
Farr, R. M. (1987), 'The science of mental life: A social psychological perspective', *Bulletin of The British Psychological Society*, 40, 2–17.

Farr, R. M. and Anderson, A. (1983), 'Beyond actor/observer differences in perspectives', in M. Hewstone (ed.), *Attribution Theory: Social and functional extensions*, Oxford: Blackwell.

Farr, R. M. and Moscovici, S. (1984), 'On the nature and role of representations in self's understanding of others and of self', in M. Cook (ed.), *Issues in Person Perception*, London: Methuen.

Friedman, N. (1967), *The Social Nature of Psychological Research: The psychological experiment as a social interaction*, New York: Basic Books.

Gallie, W. B. (1952), *Peirce and Pragmatics*, Harmondsworth: Penguin.

Garrod, S. and Anderson, A. (1987), 'Saying what you mean in dialogue: A study in conceptual and semantic co-ordination', *Cognition*, 27, 181–218.

Goffman, E. (1956), *The Presentation of Self in Everyday Life*, Edinburgh: University of Edinburgh Social Sciences Research Centre.

Goffman, E. (1981), *Forms of Talk*, Oxford: Blackwell.

Heider, F. (1958), *The Psychology of Interpersonal Relations*, New York: Wiley.

Ichheiser, G. (1949), 'Misunderstandings in human relations: A study in false social perception', *American Journal of Sociology*, 55(2/2), Monograph supplement, 1–70.

Jones, E. E. and Davis, K. E. (1965), 'From acts to dispositions: The attribution process in person perception', in L. Berkowitz (ed.), *Advances in Experimental Social Psychology*, vol. 2, New York: Academic Press.

Jones, E. E. and Nisbett, R. E. (1972), 'The actor and the observer: Divergent perceptions of the causes of behavior', in E. E. Jones, D. E. Kanouse, H. H. Kelley, R. E. Nisbett, S. Valins and B. Weiner (eds), *Attribution: Perceiving the causes of behavior*, Morristown, NJ: General Learning Press.

Lewin, K. (1935), *A Dynamic Theory of Personality*, New York and London: McGraw-Hill.

Marková, I. (1982), *Paradigms, Thought and Language*, Chichester: Wiley.

Marková, I. (1983), 'The origin of the social psychology of language in German expressivism', *British Journal of Social Psychology*, 22, 315–25.

Marková, I. (1987), *Human Awareness: Its social development*, London: Hutchinson.

Mead, G. H. (1904), 'The relations of psychology and philology', *Psychological Bulletin*, 1, 375–91.

Mead, G. H. (1934), *Mind, Self and Society: From the standpoint of a social behaviorist*, edited and with an introduction by C. W. Morris, Chicago: University of Chicago Press.

Meyer, M. F. (1921), *The Psychology of the Other One: An introductory textbook*, Columbia, Miss.: Missouri Book Company.

Morris, C. W. (1938), 'Foundations of the theory of signs', in O. Neurath (ed.), *International Encyclopedia of Unified Science*, vol. 1, ii, pp. 1–59, Chicago: University of Chicago Press.

Morris, C. W. (1946), *Signs, Language and Behavior*, New York: Prentice-Hall.

Newcomb, T. M. (1952), *Social Psychology*, London: Tavistock.

Newcomb, T. M. (1961), *The Acquaintance Process*, New York: Holt, Rinehart & Winston.

Newcomb, T. M. (1968), 'Interpersonal balance', in R. P. Abelson, E. Aronson, W. J. McGuire, T. M. Newcomb, M. J. Rosenberg and P. H. Tannenbaum (eds), *Theories of Cognitive Consistency: A sourcebook*, Chicago: Rand McNally.

Newcomb, T. M., Turner, R. H. and Converse, P. E. (1965), *Social Psychology: A study of human interaction* (revised edition), New York: Holt, Rinehart & Winston.

Rommetveit, R. (1968), *Words, Meanings and Messages*, New York: Academic Press.

Rommetveit, R. (1974), *On Message Structure: A framework for the study of language and communication*, New York: Wiley.

Rommetveit, R. (1984), 'The role of language in the creation and transmission of social representations', in R. M. Farr and S. Moscovici (eds), *Social Representations*, Cambridge: Cambridge University Press.

Ross, L. (1977), 'The intuitive psychologist and his shortcomings: Distortions in the attribution process', in L. Berkowitz (ed.), *Advances in Experimental Social Psychology*, vol. 10, New York: Academic Press.

Simmel, G. (1955a), *Conflict*, trans. K. H. Wolff, New York: Glencoe.

Simmel, G. (1955b), *The Web of Group Affiliations*, trans. R. Bendix, New York: Glencoe.

Skinner, B. F. (1957), *Verbal Behavior*, New York: Appleton-Century-Crofts.

Watson, J. B. (1925), *Behaviorism*, New York: Norton.

Wundt, W. (1900–20), *Völkerpsychologie: Eine Untersuchung der Entwicklungsgesetze von Sprache, Mythos und Sitte*, 10 vols, Leipzig: Engelmann.

Wundt, W. (1916), *Elements of Folk Psychology: Outlines of a psychological history of the development of mankind*, trans. L. Schaub, London: George Allen & Unwin.

Wundt, W. (1973), *The Language of Gestures*, with an introduction by A. L. Blumenthal and additional essays on G. H. Mead and K. Bühler. The Hague: Mouton.

2 | Social communication, dialogue and conversation

Thomas Luckmann
Department of Sociology, University of Konstanz

On the genetic aspects of social communication

It may be useful to begin by defining the key concepts of this chapter. In general accordance with the etymology of the word, 'dialogue' may be taken to mean social communication of a particular kind which is based on language. 'Language' is understood here in a precise rather than a metaphorically extended sense: as a system of signs rather than merely signals. Thus, by definition, dialogue is a universal component of human life *and*, at the same time, it is limited to our species. Social communication by means other than a fully developed language is of course much older than dialogue and may be assumed to characterize social interaction between individuated organisms of all species.

To the extent that we adhere to *some* evolutionist notion of the origin of the varied forms of life, we must assume that dialogue could not but have emerged from more primitive forms of social communication. This point, obvious as it may be, is sufficiently important for successive generations of scholars and scientists engaged in the study of language to have continued to ponder its implications. Looking merely at the last fifty or sixty years (roughly the time span separating contemporary theory from G. H. Mead's (1934, p. 63) analysis of the 'conversation of gestures' in the genealogy of 'mind', and Vygotsky's interactionist, sociological position in his debate with Piaget), we see that considerable progress has been made in following up important implications of this general point in ontogenetic contexts (Bruner, 1978; Tronik, Als and Adamson, 1979; Trevarthen and Hubley, 1978; Trevarthen, 1979; Dore, 1978). If one says that the dialogue of a child develops from pre-linguistic social communication, two things are presupposed. The first is that the child is equipped with the potential for pre-linguistic reciprocity.[1] The second is that language is a communicative resource which represents a socio-historical a priori both for the child learning to talk and for its mother who herself was a child at one time, first participating in an 'action dialogue' (Bruner, 1978) and then in true dialogue with *her* mother. Knowledge pertaining to these two assumptions has accumulated slowly in various fields. Studies of the ontogenesis of dialogue which contributed to such knowledge were mainly inspired by the developmental approach in psycholinguistics and social psychology. There has also been some hesitant phylogenetic speculation on the 'origins' of language – for so long a taboo topic in linguistics and anthropology. Such speculation has tended to extrapolate from ethological and experimental studies of animal communication, especially the communication of primates.

The main results of these studies are well known. On the whole, they lend concrete plausibility to what, in the abstract, must in any case be taken for granted by all adherents of some sort of evolutionary logic: that language as a historical sign system evolved from pre-linguistic reciprocal communicative action. It is obvious – a consequence of the very nature of the problem – that there can be no ontogenetic parallel to the interactional phylogenesis of language. However, phylogenetic assumptions about the interactional origins of language are supported by work carried out in an entirely different area of scholarly discourse: phenomenological analyses of the 'constitution' of language show that it originates in intersubjective communication (Luckmann, 1972; 1983a). In studies limited to the *onto*genetic aspects of dialogue, the evolutionary emergence of language can be perhaps taken for granted, and language, considered as an unproblematic socio-historical a priori, can simply be inserted as a given entity into accounts of the individual's acquisition of language. In a general discussion of the origins of dialogue, however, it is not superfluous to keep in mind the general phylogenetic background of the problem, and a few systematic observations on this matter are in order.[2]

In the widest sense of the term, even the transmission of information from one cell to another may be regarded as an elementary form of 'social' communication. In a sensible restriction of the term, however, one may wish to designate as social only those kinds of communication which take place between individuated organisms. Such elementary forms of communication as genetic coding, information processing in physiological feedback systems, etc. must have been enormously important in the evolution of life forms. *Social communication* (in the strict sense of the term) may no doubt also be regarded as an adaptive process, although it is located on a more complex level of the organization of life. After that theoretical assumption is made, the interest of the social scientist turns elsewhere. Considerations of adaptation and evolution are too general and too abstract to be of much concern to the social sciences, for which time spans of a historical order of magnitude are relevant: social communication determines in a significant way the everyday conduct of the members of our species as members of historic cultures and constitutes the fabric of human social organization. Despite such reasons for considering questions of adaptation and evolution as outside the purview of the social sciences, a brief consideration of the most important general functions of social communication (sociality, reciprocity, abstraction and intentionality) may be useful, because it will show the generic background to the specifically human aspects of social communication.

Sociality refers to the regulation of communicative behaviour by means of a code. That code may be transmitted in a species either by genetic programming or by 'learning' or by a combination of the two. *Reciprocity* refers to the systematic interdependence of behaviour in which one organism's action is a response to the action of another, and vice versa. This continuous alternation of feedback from one organism to another presupposes that the ability of an individual organism to observe (and to interpret consciously or automatically) the behaviour of other individuals is imputed by that individual to others, and that, in consequence, its own behaviour is adjusted to anticipated observation (and interpretation) by them. *Abstraction* is the ability to refer in communication not only to the actual components of the communicative situation (which are thus simultaneously accessible to the participants in the communicative interaction), but also to elements which transcend that situation either in space or in time or in both. *Intentionality* refers to the awareness on the part of an individual organism of the communicative possibilities of its species, more particularly of its code or codes, and its ability either to use them selectively or to abstain from using them with a (communicative) purpose.

It is clear that in different species social communication is based on different kinds of sociality, different forms of reciprocity and unequal degrees of abstraction and intentionality. But it should be added that it is also characterized by different *combinations* of these dimensions of social communication. (Evidently, it is not necessary to assume that the evolution of these 'functions' was closely synchronized, although it is likely that their development was somehow interrelated.) For the individual members of most species, social behaviour (sociality) is programmed genetically in a rather rigid fashion; but with the mammals, and especially with the primates, it comes to depend in increasing measure upon individual experience and intersubjective learning. It is well known that abstraction is highly developed in the social communication of the honey bee, but is absent or low in that of most other species, including mammals. Significantly, the faculty for abstraction reappears with the higher primates. Intentionality, finally, has extremely complex physiological presuppositions; its adaptive value is probably linked to the individualization of social relations in certain mammal species (e.g. among chimpanzees), and it represents an evolutionarily recent acquisition in the development of life forms.

The most complex and most highly differentiated form of social communication is undoubtedly found in our species. It presupposes the evolution of flexible ('individualized') sociality, full reciprocity, high abstraction and advanced intentionality, and is based on a systematic combination of these functions. Whatever may have been the conditions for their development, it makes sense to assume that they were present in hominid evolution. However, their most advanced combination, leading to the production and transmission of a fully fledged system of social communication in the form of language, may be limited to *homo sapiens*.[3] The simultaneous presence of these highly perfected functions was undoubtedly necessary for the emergence of a communication system which was genetically 'underdetermined' and thus capable of historicization in long chains of intersubjective communicative acts.

Natural and historical systems of social communication

Human social communication based on language passed the line dividing 'natural' systems of social communication from 'historical' ones. In a metaphorical sense, history itself may be said to have emerged from nature. Since systems of social communication are products of natural selection, and since languages are the main elements of human social communication, language must be regarded as the result of evolutionary processes. Yet language is a rather peculiar system of social communication and differs from the systems of social communication of other species in a highly significant way:

even if it is a product of evolution, it is less directly so than social communication in other species. In a manner of speaking, it is the product of a product: languages, in the concrete plural, are the historical sediments of complex chains of (communicative) human *actions*.

Although language must have evolved from some more primitive system of social communication, and although, on a high level of abstraction, the functions of language may be considerd analogous to the functions of social communication in other species, this analogy does not greatly illuminate the nature of language. As an evolutionary emergent, language reaches a higher level of complexity both in function and in structure. In comparison with older forms there is a qualitative change in the method of production, transmission and use of the system of social communication. The elementary presuppositions in the human individual for the production, transmission and use of the linguistic code – these include a cognitive 'depth-structure' – continue to be genetically transmitted. They are part of the human biogram (Count, 1970, 1974). But the linguistic codes themselves, these essential elements of a socio-historical a priori, are the result of social interaction. They represent the basic stratum of the cumulative historical record of human communicative acts. The transmission of the code, too, consists of intentional communicative acts – difficult as it may be to draw a line between production and transmission. And, obviously, the ordinary everyday use of the code also consists of such intentional communicative acts.

In the formulation of theories about dialogue it must be taken into account that languages as historical systems of signs did not entirely replace the phylogenetically older elements of social communication. Thus a situation of unprecedented complexity arose. On the one hand, language became the central system of social communication, replacing whatever had served as the main code at an earlier stage. On the other hand, elements of the phylogenetically older components of social communication, most importantly those linked to gesture, posture and facial expression, continued to coexist with language. They could perform partly language-independent, partly language-dependent communicative functions.

If the original use of language shows a high degree of intentionality, the original employment of the phylogenetically older components of social communication tends to be guided by 'instinct'. But that is not the whole story. The most elementary preconditions for human communication hardly ever pass the threshold of consciousness. Furthermore, there are many conscious aspects of communication which are not unequivocally purposive – they are part of human behaviour, but they enter interaction only as raw material, if at all. Startling due to fright and outbursts of tears occur consciously, but are not planned actions. It is hard to draw a precise line between purposive and non-purposive conduct, between mere behaviour and action. For one thing, even those expressive phenomena which are basically involuntary rather than purposive, and with regard to whose occurrence in social situations there is little or no reciprocity of production and 'reception', may be consciously controlled to a certain extent so that they can be employed intentionally in social interaction.

Conversely, many components of the communicative process which were originally conscious and intentional sink back into something like secondary passivity (to us a phenomenological concept). Examples of such transformations range from physical performances (such as the mouth position for the proper pronunciation of a consonant) to interpretive accomplishments involved in the understanding of the meaning of a sentence. Through frequent repetition such communicative activities may become fully routinized. None the less, they are not to be equated with the phylogenetically early, *originally* automatic processes.

This point that communication which originally was conscious and intentional tends by frequent repetition to become routinized, shows that the line dividing those phenomena in which our 'naturalness' is still clearly discernible, from those in which a social-historical sign system (most commonly language) is purposively applied, is blurred. Generally one may observe that in face-to-face communication the use of language recombines with the partly instinctive, partly intentional employment of other means of social communication.

The complex possibilities of human social communication can increase when, analogously with the development of a linguistic code, abstract codes based on other than the vocal modality become possible. These may serve as substitutes for the main code – as does, for example, American Sign Language for the deaf – or they may be used in addition to it in special situations.

The immediate antecedents of languages as historical sign systems were probably rather rudimentary proto-linguistic communicative codes which arose from uncodified or weakly codified social communication. The beginnings of the social *construction* of communicative codes must be traced back to a stage in which phylogenetically older elements of social communication could be used with considerable flexibility and in which, concurrently, highly individualized social interaction was possible. Highly individualized social interaction is characterized by full reciprocity and thus allows for effective *intersubjective mirroring*.[4] In such interactions those elements which are (potentially) relevent to the other participants in the situation can be communicated to them by typical expressive forms of a vocal, gestural, postural and mimetic nature. Most importantly, the expressive forms can be reproduced in the anticipation of a typical, recurrent interpretation (reception) by others. And the production by one individual can be imitated by others. Under these circumstances it seems plausible to assume that the most important items of *intersubjective* relevance are *subjective action* projects which play a role in the coordination of social action.

In the early stages of the development of language, in the phylogenetic and ontogenetic senses, to have any chance of success communicative acts had to refer to objects and events in the common reach of the participants in the communicative situation. In other words, communication was embedded in deixis. Traces of this are left in all languages (Benveniste, 1971; Tur-Sinai, 1957). This limitation was overcome after the faculty of abstraction and the sign-linked ability to remember reached a certain level. (The emergence of this level need not have been directly and exclusively linked to social communication; another important factor may have been the adaptive value of certain kinds of generalization for subjective memory and the planning of individual action.) In the process of intersubjective mirroring, the production of expressive forms becomes standardized. This means that the interpretation of the subjective meaning of an expressive form for its producer, the subjective interpretation of it by the addressee and the subjective anticipation of this interpretation (by the addressee) on the part of the producer become congruent for all practical purposes (Luckmann, 1972). Thus, once again in the 'evolution' of codes of social communication, a relatively fixed code is established – with the difference, on this occasion, that the code is used *intentionally* by the participants in communicative processes as members of historical linguistic communities. In the full reciprocity of the communicative situation, with an increase in the degree of abstraction and growing intentional control of production and interpretation of expressive forms, deixis becomes less and less important. Contextual ellipsis become possible. In other words, communicative acts may eventually refer to elements of the world of everyday life, shared by speaker and listener, which transcend the communicative situation in space and time. At that point expressive forms turn into proto-signs.

It is a matter of interactional economy as well as an element of the generation contract (to appropriate a term from a different context), that the relation between the *significans* and the *significatum* be made obligatory. Once this had happened in the development of social communication, the proto-signs became signs in the full sense of the word. In the absence of a genetically fixed communicative code (with all the disadvantages caused by the rigidity of genetic programming) the congruence of meaning in encoding and decoding was of course a matter of extreme importance. It was the presupposition for the routinized intentional functioning of social communication, and must have been subject to social control, and therefore power, from the beginning. Thus the intersubjective construction of proto-signs, although reciprocal, was asymmetrical. The elements of the communicative code acquired full sign status as soon as social control was exercised in the *transmission* of the elements of the code to others, especially to another generation.

Whether one tries to understand the genetic aspect of dialogue or its interactional dynamics, it is important to keep in mind that whereas the basic conditions and the elementary constituents of the human system of social communication are the result of human phylogenesis, the main code of human social communication is an evolutionary emergent and is socially constructed in history.

Dialogue in face-to-face interaction

If one compares the various forms of human communication, it is evident that dialogue is the elementary form and that the others are, in one way or another, derivative.[5] Indeed, several dialogical features appear to be primitive. This is due to the situational embeddedness of the dialogical communicative process, and to the fact that dialogue is always concretely actualized as part of face-to-face social interaction. No matter how 'well formed' dialogue is linguistically, and no matter how far removed its topics are from the concrete aspects of the situation in which it takes place, it continues to exhibit traces of its primitive, pre-linguistic origin.

Among all the forms of language use, dialogue is characterized by the highest degree of immediacy and reciprocity. Persons participating in dialogue are in the presence of one another, they are in the unique position of sharing time and space with one another. Sharing a sector of the world is a prerequisite for mutual attention and a condition for what Alfred Schutz called the synchronization of two streams of consciousness (Schutz, 1932/1973). With the aid of notational systems (such as writing), reciprocal sign-bound communication is also possible *without* the synchronization of two streams of consciousness. However, the reciprocity involved in that instance is evidently delayed rather than immediate. On the other hand, synchronization of two streams of consciousness may of course also occur without sign-related communication. Dialogue, however, presupposes both sign-bound communication – which rests upon a sign system, a code – and the synchronization of two streams of consciousness. In consequence, dialogue is both logos and concrete, embodied intersubjectivity. It is not surprising, therefore, that it is normally highly deictic and sensitive to the extra-linguistic and non-communicative components of the situation. (If this situational sensitivity is to be reduced, special provisions must be made against it, as in formal etiquettes, ritual exclusions, etc.)[6] In short, every dialogue is embedded in 'action dialogue'.

The presence of the other for each of the participants in a dialogue has systematic rather than merely fortuitous consequences for the linguistic aspects of the dialogue. The code-constituted autonomy of meaning (i.e. the signification of the word) in a dialogue is limited.[7] This is not only an 'objective' fact perceived by an analytically minded observer; it is also a circumstance well known to the participants in dialogue. Speakers are vaguely – and, on occasion, even precisely – aware of a common core of meaning of a word in different contexts of use. They are also aware of the communicative (and interactional) purpose of what they are saying when they use that word at a particular time to a particular listener. When engaged in a dialogue, they follow the principle of the reciprocity of perspectives in assuming, until further notice, that the listener listens – and speaks – on the basis of similar understandings. Against the background of mutual attention (in which, as was stated above, the synchronization of two steams of consciousness comes about) everything that is said is interpretable as *situated* action. In other words, it is interpretable first and foremost not as an abstract message or as a sentence, but as something that the speaker intends, and says to this particular interlocutor here and now, as an utterance.[8]

Furthermore, everything that is said in a dialogue is articulated by the speaker in reasonable awareness of the communicative possibilities of non-verbal modalities and in corresponding awareness that the listener knows of the speaker's awareness of such communicative possibilities and thus imputes to him or her a certain degree of choice when he or she makes use of one of these possibilities rather than another. The signification of what is said is embedded in the interactional meaning of what (*hic et nunc*) is *not* said, and in the meaning of *how* it is said. A word is not merely emphasized by gestures, nor is it only illustrated by facial expressions. The full meaning of a 'statement' in a dialogue is produced systematically by combining the code-derived, anonymized, idealized and relatively stable signification of the syntactic–semantic–phonetic options of language (Halliday, 1973). These options are chosen, or routinely employed, by the speaker, along with body-postures, gestures and facial expressions which are laden with particular meanings.

Such combined communicative actions are, of course, never self-enclosed soliloquies. Rather, they are typical, more or less planned, more or less routinized, combined verbal/non-verbal productions. Both the content and the form of the communicative productions are co-determined by anticipations of typical receptions. Such anticipations are either part of the conscious production plan or are imprinted in the production by frequent repetition.[9] The principle of 'recipient design' in oral communication has been described in conversational analysis by, e.g., Sacks, Schegloff and Jefferson (1974, p. 727) and Sacks and Schegloff (1979). It is, first of all, an element in the planning, and the routines, of everyday linguistic communicative acts. But it is more than that: it is also constitutive of a unitary, multi-modal communicative *praxis*.

Indubitably, *everything* that a participant does in face-to-face communication may be taken to indicate something about him or her. But there is an important difference between what is attributable to him or her as a producer, as a normally competent participant in dialogue, and what is not. Involuntarily emitted sounds can be embarrassing, a change of complexion betraying. Although such 'communicative events' are mere events rather than communicative 'productions', they are certainly relevant for the interpretation of a participant's activities by other participants. However, contingent aspects of behaviour (or aspects which can be made to seem contingent by behavioural procedures which Goffman (1981) described with great precision) which haphazardly enter the production of signification in dialogue are also typically received as contingent. On the other hand, anything in the communicative process that typically *can* be produced on purpose is habitually interpreted as a component of dialogue by the participants – whether it was in fact consciously produced in a particular instance or not. Such interpretations can, however, be modified or nullified by the involuntary (or, as one must be careful to add, pseudo-involuntary) producer by his or her engaging in specific 'repair actions' (Schegloff, Jefferson and Sacks, 1977).

Despite the systematic multimodality of dialogue, actions and interpretations of communicative actions tend to be centred upon the verbal dimension. This is fairly obviously the case in modern Western societies, but it may not be equally so in societies which are not characterized by such a highly verbalized form of communicative culture as ours. The core of the planning of communicative acts at least in Western societies is speech planning with a syntactic–semantic focus. The non-linguistic expressive components tend to be less purposively planned, and those that are purposive tend to be more highly routinized. An obvious exception must be made for professional actors, and in all societies there are probably also some non-professionals who 'instinctively' master higher arts of expression management. In addition, a certain amount of coaching by professionals may replace 'instinct'.[10]

It is well documented that in many non-Western societies attention to *non*-linguistic aspects of communicative processes is more highly developed than in ours. (There are many anecdotes about the difficulties, embarrassments and comic situations which result from this circumstance in intercultural encounters.) A growing body of research and observation has shown that in our societies, too, there are, or were, class-specific and regional variations in the communicative culture. Among other things, a communicative culture is characterized by a specific mixture of the verbal and non-verbal components of dialogue. Cultural, historical and class variations in these are very probably linked to the oral/literary cultural syndrome, to the nature of the dominant institutions of socialization (family, school, etc.) and, more generally, to the communicative 'budget' of a society with its characteristic repertoire of communicative genres – and the social distribution of that repertoire.

Dialogue and conversation

At the beginning of this chapter I made the assumption that dialogue is a human universal. Now we must examine whether this is merely an arbitrary terminological proposal or whether, rather, it is a hypothesis of some substance. Does one want to use the term 'dialogue' in the most general sense, thereby subsuming under it certain universal components of human communication? (This is the sense in which I have used it so far.) Or does one wish to restrict the use of the term to the specific case of just one of a multitude of different historical forms of communication? It may seem that what is at issue is merely the merits of one terminological decision over another. As is often the case, however, concept and substance are closely connected. One must guard against the danger that the choice of a particular term directs theoretical attention to one level of the phenomena of human communication, to the detriment of interest in other levels.

In my view a stronger terminological case can be made for the first rather than the second alternative. Dialogue as a universal form of human communication can be defined with considerable precision in a purely formal way: dialogue is sign-bound face-to-face communication which involves that high degree of immediacy and reciprocity which occurs when the streams of consciousness of the participants in social communication are fully synchronized. The term thus refers to the most elementary form of human communication. But the definition of dialogue in such formal terms is merely the first step. Two additional questions immediately arise. First, are there additional attributes of dialogue which are also universal? Or, second, are there certain substantive features which characterize concrete historical variants of dialogue and which are limited to some periods or a few cultures only? A third question follows upon these two: is dialogue, defined in formal terms, necessarily realized in specific historical variants with changing substantive features?

In the search for universal attributes of dialogue, *equality* has most frequently been thought to qualify, especially in philosophical discourse. It seems obvious, however, that something like *power* (tending to produce *in*equality), rather than something like equality, commonly characterizes social face-to-face communication, not only in other species but also in our own.[11] Equality, therefore, will not do as a universal and defining characteristic of dialogue. What about the possibility, though, that something like equality has come to characterize a particular *historical* variant of dialogue?

Provisionally we may assume that under certain circumstances in some, if not in all, societies and cultures, a specific form of dialogue emerges which is characterized by equality. Communicative situations in which the partners are equal occur in archaic, traditional and modern societies, in those which are only weakly stratified through kin relations and in those which are hierarchically ordered in castes, estates or social classes. That much seems certain – but of course it is also trivial with regard to our problem. When social equality is carried *into* dialogue, in other words, when it is established *beforehand* through status-symmetry of the participants in social communication, it is not an immanent structural aspect of dialogue. Dialogue characterized by such extraneous equality may be observable as a specific, socio-structurally determined and historically limited variant of dialogue. But evidently it is not a general feature of dialogical, face-to-face communication.

However, the existence of communicative equality as a consequence of *antecedent* social equality does not logically exclude the possibility of an intrinsically *communicative* equality which may emerge from some essential features of dialogue. This possibility deserves consideration. On the one hand there exist status inequality and communicative asymmetry. On the other hand, equality is imported, as it were, into a communicative situation by antecedent status definitions. Quite apart from these phenomena, is there not something in the very nature of dialogue which in all societies imposes a temporary and provisional enactment of an 'as-if-equality' *whenever* the social structure does not compellingly impose inequality upon the communicative process? Social inequality generally tends to impose communicative asymmetry in strongly institutionalized social interaction. There are few traditionally institutionalized forms of dialogical communication which show equality or, to put matters in a neutral fashion, symmetry. In confessions of guilt, consultation between social workers and clients, sales talks, etc., little more by way of symmetry can be found than that which can be traced to the elementary dialogical attribute of reciprocity. It is not implausible to assume, however, that in the absence of strong institutional constraints, intentional reciprocity may produce a kind of temporary symmetry between the participants in dialogue which goes beyond reciprocity itself and which may be experienced and practised as a kind of as-if-equality. If this assumption is correct, as I think it is, we may find it useful to distinguish between dialogue as a universal and elementary form of human communication, and different kinds of historical, socio-structurally and culturally limited subspecies of dialogue. Among these, the subspecies which we call conversation is of particular interest because it shows how the inherent possibility of reciprocity turning temporarily into equality can emerge as an actual historical genre.

No doubt we touch here upon a matter which was, and still is, ideologically contaminated. This area of discourse has always been subject to different social constructions and widely divergent religious and theoretical interpretations. Various forms and degrees of power and helplessness, dominance and inferiority are brought into the processes of conversation from 'the outside', from 'society', whether they are accentuated in a given culture or denied ideologically. More importantly, from the present point of view, the phenomena of power and dominance also appear in conversation itself. They emerge, at the very least, as a sediment of the sequence of communicative acts.[12] In sum, the equality which characterizes conversation as a subspecies of dialogue is highly vulnerable not only from the outside but also from within.

Tentatively, we may define conversation as a historical subspecies of dialogue in which a relatively high degree of specifically communicative symmetry, typically experienced as equality, prevails. Conversation, I add here without further elaboration, is a multifunctional and weakly institutionalized communicative process and would not qualify under most definitions of genre (except perhaps in the very wide one proposed by Bakhtin, 1986). In spite of the above definition, the possibility of different functional priorities in different historical variants of conversation should not be excluded a priori from consideration. One should also keep in mind that under historically unusual circumstances, even equality may become institutionalized as the ideal form of dialogue as, for example, in scientific discourse, and it may become a constitutive feature of specific dialogical genres.

Conclusion

Dialogue may thus be taken to refer to the elementary and universal form of human communication which is genetically determined by the joint development of individualized sociality, reciprocity, abstraction and intentionality. The dialogical process is based on the concrete, situationally embedded (face-to-face) synchronization of two (or more) streams of consciousness *and* the use of language (or another quasi-ideal historical sign system) as the dominant medium of communication. Conversation, on the other hand, refers to a range of historical subspecies of dialogue which, in contradistinction to various other dialogical subspecies, are characterized by a tendency toward intrinsic (communicative) equality of the participants – typically under conditions of relatively weak social–structural (institutionalized) constraints upon the communicative situation (unless, exceptionally, communicative equality itself is institutionalized), as well as by multimodality and polyfunctionality of the communicative process.

Dialogues, in the sense understood here, evidently contain the oldest layers of human communication which, for their part, retain essential characteristics of the phylogenetically older still 'action dialogue'. At the same time, dialogues are also specifically human inasmuch as they involve the purposive use of a historical sign system. The term 'conversation', on the other hand, is employed here in a way which directs attention to broad similarities in certain historical subspecies of the elementary and universal structures of dialogue.

If these concepts are theoretically useful, it should be possible to distinguish in empirical analyses two genetically distinct but interpenetrating layers of oral communication: the old and elementary dialogical substrate and a superimposed younger historical level, for example, a conversational one. If the assumption that the former is universal is correct, structural features of the elementary level should be found in all texts (i.e. transcripts) of oral communication. Which of these features will characterize a given text is a matter for further consideration and much comparative empirical analysis. It may be that conversational forms make up a limited, but perhaps nevertheless fairly wide, range of cultural and social variation in dialogical communication. Whether or not conversation is a distinctive genre of oral communication (and if so, where and how) is another question, one which deserves systematic attention.[13]

Notes

1. Trevarthen and others studying eye contact between babies and mothers have shown that this potential begins to be realized earlier than was commonly supposed and Bruner and others traced the development of dialogue in an elementary 'action dialogue' (Trevarthen and Hubley, 1978; Trevarthen, 1979; Bruner, 1978).
2. I sketched this background in 'Language in society' (Luckmann, 1984b). The main part of the first section of this chapter is based on that and some formulations are taken from it. From the voluminous literature on the subject I shall mention here just a few: Count, 1974; Hockett, 1960; Lieberman, 1972; Jolly, 1972.
3. For a brief bibliographical documentation of these general observations, see Luckmann, 1983a, 1983b.
4. For the 'discovery' of the 'looking glass' effect, see Cooley, 1902/1964 and Mead, 1934/1967. This effect is the intersubjective foundation of the social construction of personal identity.
5. For an earlier version of these observations, see my 'Das Gespräch' (Luckmann, 1984a).
6. See Bergmann, this volume, Chapter 9.
7. Vološinov, 1929/1973 was not facetious when he wrote that, strictly speaking, signification (meaning) does not signify (mean) anything. His distinction between meaning and theme is paralleled by Bakhtin's (1986) distinction between sentence and utterance. These positions are echoes – and specifications – of Humboldt's famous point that language is both *ergon* and *energeia* (1836).
8. Remember Bakhtin's discussion of the interactional context of utterances.

   But in reality any communication like that, addressed to someone or evoking something, has a particular purpose, that is, it is a real link in the chain of speech communion in a particular sphere of human activity or everyday life. (1986, p.83)

9. These terms are adapted from recent aesthetic theory of literary production and 'reception' (Jauss, 1977/1982 and Iser, 1972/1974).

10. For a detailed analysis of these matters in modern politics see Atkinson, 1984.
11. For a careful discussion of the issues involved here see Linell, 1979.
12. See Linell, 1979.
13. Starting from earlier work (Luckmann, 1989a) I addressed this question in my contribution to the *Festschrift for Ragnar Rommetveit* (Luckmann, 1989b).

References

Atkinson, J. M. (1984), *Our Masters' Voices: The language and body language of politics*, London and New York: Methuen.
Bakhtin, M. M. (1986), *Speech Genres and Other Late Essays*, Austin, Texas: University of Texas Press.
Benveniste, E. (1971), *Problems in General Linguistics*, Coral Gables, Fla.: University of Miami Press.
Bruner, J. S. (1978), 'Acquiring the uses of language' (Berlyne Memorial Lecture), *Canadian Journal of Psychology* (Revue Canad. Psychol.) 32, 204–18.
Cooley, C. H. (1902/1964), *Human Nature and the Social Order*, New York: Schocken.
Count, E. W. (1970), *Das Biogramm. Anthropologische Studien*, Frankfurt: Fischer.
Count, E. W. (1974), 'On the phylogenesis of the speech function', *Current Anthropology*, 15, 81–8.
Dore, J. (1978), 'Conditions for the acquisition of speech acts', in I. Marková (ed.), *The Social Context of Language*, Chichester and New York: Wiley.
Goffman, E. (1981), *Forms of Talk*, Oxford: Blackwell.
Halliday, M. A. K. (1973), *Explorations in the Functions of Language*, London: Arnold.
Hockett, C. F. (1960), 'The origin of speech', *Scientific American*, 203, 3–10.
Humboldt, W. von (1836), *Üeber die Verschiedenheit des menschlichen Sprachbaues*, Berlin.
Iser, W. (1972/1974), *Der implizite Leser: Kommunikationsformen des Romans von Bunyan bis Beckett*, München: Fink, trans. as *The Implied Reader: Patterns of communication in prose-fiction from Bunyan to Beckett*, Baltimore: Johns Hopkins University Press.
Jauss, H. R. (1977/1982), *Aesthetische Erfahrung und literarische Hermeneutik*, München: Fink, trans. as *Aesthetic Experience and Literary Hermeneutics*, Minneapolis: University of Minnesota Press.
Jolly, A. (1972), *The Evolution of Primate Behavior*, New York and Toronto: The Macmillan Co.
Lieberman, P. (1972), *The Speech of Primates*, The Hague and Paris: Mouton.
Linell, P. (1979), *Psychological Reality in Phonology: A theoretical study*, Cambridge: Cambridge University Press.
Luckmann, T. (1972), 'The constitution of language in the world of everyday life', in L. E. Embree (ed.), *Life-World and Consciousness: Essay for Aron Gurwitsch*, Evanston, Ill.: Northwestern University Press.
Luckmann, T. (1983a), 'Elements of a social theory of communication', in Luckmann, *Life-World and Social Realities*, London: Heinemann Educa-

tional Books (originally in: H. P. Althaus *et al.* (eds), *Lexikon der Germanistischen Linguistik*, Tübingen 1973, (1979²)).
Luckmann, T. (1983b), 'Personal identity as an evolutionary and historical problem', in Luckmann, *Life-World and Social Realities*, London: Heinemann Educational Books (originally in: Cranach, M. von, Foppa, K., Lepenies, W. and Ploog, D. (eds) (1979), *Human Ethology: Claims and limits of a new discipline*, Cambridge: Cambridge University Press.
Luckmann, T. (1984a), 'Das Gespräch', in K. Stierle and R. Warning (eds.) *Das Gespräch* (Poetik und Hermeneutik XI), München: Fink.
Luckmann, T. (1984b), 'Language in society', *International Social Science Journal*, 36, 5–20.
Luckmann, T. (1989a), 'Communicative genres in the communicative "budget" of a society' (lecture, University of Oslo, May 1985), to be published in an adapted version with the title 'Prolegomena to a social theory of communicative genres: In memory of Toussaint Hocevar', forthc. in A. Lokar (ed.), *Essays in Memory of Toussaint Hocevar*, special issue of *Slovene Studies*, 1989.
Luckmann, T. (1989b), 'Conversation and communicative genres', forthc. in Heen Wold (ed.) *Festschrift for Ragnar Rommetveit*.
Mead, G. H. (1934/1967), *Mind, Self and Society*, Chicago: University of Chicago Press.
Sacks, H. and Schegloff, E. A. (1979), 'Two preferences in the organization of reference to persons in conversation and their interaction', in G. Psathas (ed.), *Everyday Language: Studies in ethnomethodology*, New York: Irvington.
Sacks, H., Schegloff, E. A., Jefferson, G. (1974), 'A simplest systematics for the organization of turn-taking for conversation', *Language*, 50, 696–735.
Schegloff, E. A., Jefferson, G. and Sacks, H. (1977), 'The preference for self-correction in the organization of repair in conversation', *Language*, 53, 361–82.
Schutz, A. (1932/1973), *Der Sinnhafte Aufbau der Sozialen Welt. Eine Einleitung in die verstehende Soziologie*, Wien: Springer; trans. by R. M. Zaner and H. T. Engelhardt as *The Phenomenology of the Social World*, Evanston, Ill.: Northwestern University Press, 1973 (second edition); London: Heinemann (1974).
Trevarthen, C. (1979), 'Instincts for human understanding and for cultural cooperation: Their development in infancy', in: Cranach, M. von, Foppa, K., Lepenies, W. and Ploog, D. (eds) (1979), *Human Ethology: Claims and limits of a new discipline*, Cambridge: Cambridge University Press.
Trevarthen, C. and Hubley, P. (1978), 'Secondary intersubjectivity: Confidence, confiding and acts of meaning in the first year', in A. Lock (ed.), *Action, Gesture and Symbol: The emergence of language*, London: Academic Press.
Tronick, E., Als, H. and Adamson, L. (1979), 'Structure of early face-to-face communicative interactions', in M. Bullowa (ed.), *Before Speech: The beginning of interpersonal communication*, Cambridge: Cambridge University Press.
Tur-Sinai, N. H. (1957), 'The origin of language', in R. N. Anshen (ed.), *Language: An enquiry into its meaning and function*, New York: Harper & Row.
Vološinov, V. N. (1929/1973), *Marxism and the Philosophy of Language*, New York and London, Seminar Press (originally: *Marksizm i filosofija jazyka*, Leningrad 1929¹).

3. Dialogue and dialogism in a socio-cultural approach to mind

James V. Wertsch
Frances L. Hiatt School of Psychology, Clark University

A socio-cultural approach to mind seeks to explicate mental processes in a way that recognizes their inherent cultural, historical and institutional situatedness. For example, a socio-cultural analysis might be concerned with the mental functioning of a modern Japanese technician, a nineteenth-century Russian aristocrat, or a North American child in a modern classroom. Socio-cultural approaches to mind have typically involved comparisons between traditional and modern societies, but they need not do so; indeed, they need not involve explicit comparison at all. The main criterion they must meet is that mental functioning be examined from a perspective that explicates how it reflects and shapes the cultural, historical and institutional setting in which it occurs.

In the past, studies that would qualify as socio-cultural approaches to mind have usually been carried out by scholars from anthropology, history, comparative sociology, cross-cultural psychology and other such disciplines. In my view, one need not be a card-carrying member of any of these disciplines to conduct such analyses. Indeed, anyone interested in psychological processes, with the possible exception of neurological functioning (but see Luria, 1971; Mecacci, 1979), is inherently concerned with socio-cultural situatedness. The point is not that we should create a new discipline to study this; instead, we

---

The writing of this chapter was assisted by the Spencer Foundation. The statements made and the views expressed are solely the responsibility of the author.

should recognize ways in which current research is implicitly grounded in assumptions about socio-culturally specific settings.

There is a wide range of methods and theoretical constructs available for studying socio-culturally situated mental processes. The approach I shall present is grounded in the assumption about the 'centrality of symbolic social communication' outlined by Marková in her Introduction to this volume (p. 3). It assumes that the study of symbolic (or what I shall term 'semiotically mediated') social communication can provide essential insights into the nature of mental processes and the embeddedness of these processes in cultural, historical and institutional settings.

A key to mapping out this approach is what I shall term 'dialogicality'. Dialogicality is a notion drawn from the writings of M. M. Bakhtin and it covers a wide range of semiotic phenomena. Its basic assumption is that spoken and written utterances can be adequately interpreted only if their interrelationships with other utterances are taken into consideration. As I shall employ it, dialogicality is a general term that concerns issues which fall under the heading both of dialogue and dialogism as outlined by Marková (this volume, Introduction). That is, it deals both with 'face-to-face interaction between two or more persons using a system of signs' (page 1) and with 'an epistemological approach to the study of mind and language as historical and cultural phenomena' (page 4).

Vygotsky's contribution to a socio-cultural approach

Much of the foundation for the socio-cultural approach I shall outline comes from the writings of the Soviet psychologist and semiotician L. S. Vygotsky (1896–1934). Vygotsky lived and worked at a time when the young people of his generation were dedicated to helping carry out the first grand experiment in socialism. This led him and his colleagues to be particularly concerned with the mental functioning that was thought to be unique to this environment. In Vygotsky's case this emerged in the form of a concern with the types of mental functioning (e.g. formal schooling and literacy) that would be essential for building the modern industrial state (Wertsch and Youniss, 1987). In some cases, this focus on formal schooling and literacy led him to restrict his approach so that he temporarily lost sight of his more general theoretical goals (Wertsch, 1985a, Introduction), a fact that has given rise to the distinction between Vygotsky the methodologist (i.e. theorist or metatheorist) and Vygotsky the psychologist

(Davydov and Radzikhovskii, 1985). While much of what I shall have to say here is concerned with the ideas of Vygotsky the psychologist, I shall try to keep the major focus on the broader set of theoretical issues that concern Vygotsky the methodologist.

Vygotsky's theoretical vision can be outlined in terms of three general themes that run throughout his writings:

1. A reliance on a genetic, or developmental method.
2. The claim that higher (i.e. uniquely human) mental functioning in the individual has its origins in social activity.
3. The claim that a defining property of human mental action is its mediation by tools ('technical tools') and signs ('psychological tools').

In all three cases, these themes were grounded in part in Vygotsky's concern with the 'methodological problem' (Zinchenko and Smirnov, 1983) of translating Marxist social theory into psychological theory. In addition, however, they were heavily influenced by the ideas of other psychologists, semioticians and philosophers. As I have noted elsewhere (Wertsch, 1985a, Introduction), the key to understanding Vygotsky's ideas about these three themes is to understand the joint influence of Marx's and others' ideas. I shall discuss each of these themes in turn below.

Genetic method

Vygotsky's genetic analysis takes as its basic premise the slogan of one of his Soviet colleagues, Blonskii (1921), that 'behaviour can be understood only as the history of behaviour'. In Vygotsky's view a genetic method is essential for answering most questions about the nature of mental functioning.

> To encompass in research the process of a given thing's development in all its phases and changes – from birth to death – fundamentally means to discover its nature, its essence, for 'it is only in movement that a body shows that it is'. Thus, the historical study of behavior is not an auxiliary aspect of theoretical study, but rather forms its very base. (Vygotsky, 1978, p. 65)

The term 'historical' here should not be equated with ontogenetic. Vygotsky was concerned with several 'genetic domains' (Wertsch, 1985b) and was particularly interested in how processes in each of them interact in the formation of mental processes. For example, in several of his writings he noted the similarities and dissimilarities between ontogenesis and phylogenesis, grounding many of his comments in Köhler's findings from ape studies (Köhler, 1927). In this connection, his major focus was on the 'natural line of development' that gives rise to 'elementary mental functioning' and how this contrasts with the 'social line of development' associated with 'higher mental functioning' which is unique to humans (*ibid.*). In contrast to phylogenesis, where a form of the natural line of development alone was supposedly in operation, ontogenesis is fundamentally characterized in Vygotsky's view by the interconnected functioning of the natural and social lines.

A genetic domain that was of greater concern to Vygotsky than phylogenesis was socio-cultural history. His comments about this domain played such a central role in his writings that in the Soviet Union his approach has come to be known as 'socio-historical' or 'cultural-historical' (Smirnov, 1975). Motivated by issues in historical materialism, he was especially interested in the different forms of mental processes that characterize distinct socio-economic epochs. It was this interest that led Vygotsky and his colleague Luria to conduct a series of what they considered to be cross-historical studies of Central Asia in the early 1930s (Luria, 1976).

Besides phylogenesis, socio-cultural history and ontogenesis, Vygotsky was interested in one additional genetic arena that is sometimes termed 'microgenesis' (Zinchenko and Gordon, 1981). There were two types of microgenetic processes that interested him. First, he was concerned with the unfolding of a single psychological act (e.g. forming a percept); second, he was concerned with the developmental transitions that occur over the course of a training or experimental session. He did not write at length about these two forms of microgenesis, but he did outline examples and recognize them as separate genetic domains. With regard to the first form, his comments about the transition from thought to word in *Thinking and Speech* (Vygotsky, 1987, Chapter 7) are instructive; in the case of the second form of microgenesis, his interest was in the development involved in training subjects in accordance with prescribed criteria before beginning an experiment (e.g. Vygotsky, 1978).

Social origins of mental functioning in the individual

The second theme that runs throughout Vygotsky's writings is the claim that higher mental functioning in the individual has its origins in social activity. Just as he argued for the necessity of studying all mental functioning from a developmental perspective, he argued that an adequate account of individual functioning must be grounded in social processes. From the earliest period in his career as a psychologist he argued that 'the social dimension of consciousness is primary in time and fact. The individual dimension of consciousness is derivative and secondary' (Vygotsky, 1979, p. 30). Many years after Vygotsky's death, Luria (1981) argued that Vygotsky's position on this issue continued to be so 'novel' as to sound paradoxical to many psychologists. As Luria noted:

> In order to explain the highly complex forms of human consciousness one must go beyond the human organism. One must seek the origins of conscious activity and 'categorical' behavior not in the recesses of the human brain or in the depths of the spirit, but in the external conditions of life. Above all, this means that one must seek these origins in the external processes of social life, in the social and historical forms of human existence. (*ibid.*, p. 25)

Vygotsky was concerned with the ways in which this general claim applies to several genetic domains, but his primary emphasis when trying to understand its implications was on ontogenesis. A general formulation of this theme in connection with ontogenesis can be found in his 'general genetic law of cultural development' (Vygotsky, 1981a).

> Any function in the child's cultural development appears twice, or on two planes. First it appears on the social plane, and then on the psychological plane. First it appears between people as an interpsychological category, and then within the child as an intrapsychological category. This is equally true with regard to voluntary attention, logical memory, the formation of concepts, and the development of volition. We may consider this position as a law in the full sense of the word, but it goes without saying that internalization transforms the process itself and changes its structure and functions. Social relations or relations among people genetically underlie all higher functions and their interrelationships. (*ibid.*, p. 163)

In this formulation of the social origins of mental functioning in the individual Vygotsky was not simply arguing that mental functioning in the individual grows out of social experience. He was making the much stronger claim that the *same* mental function can be carried out both on the interpsychological and on the intrapsychological planes.

Furthermore, he was arguing that many of the processes and structures that appear on the interpsychological plane characterize intrapsychological functioning. With regard to the properties of dialogue, this claim emerged quite pointedly in Vygotsky's writings. He argued in his account of the internalization of speech that such speech 'grows out of its social foundations by means of transferring social, collaborative forms of behavior to the sphere of the individual's psychological functioning' (Vygotsky, 1934, p. 45). This is not to say that intrapsychological functioning is some kind of simple copy of interpsychological functioning. His comments about the transformations involved in internalization warn against any such view. It does mean, however, that functioning on the two planes is viewed as being linked in an essential way by a set of genetic transitions.

Vygotsky's ideas on this issue presuppose an understanding of notions such as thinking, memory and cognition that differs fundamentally from that normally found in psychology. In his view the terms can be properly predicated of dyads and other groups as well as of individuals. This stands in contrast to the usage of these terms in contemporary psychology, where they are automatically assumed to apply to the individual only. In this latter tradition, if one wishes to extend the terms to social processes some overt marker must be employed, as in *'socially distributed* cognition' (Hutchins, forthcoming) or *'collective* memory' (Middleton, 1987).

Vygotsky's assumptions on this point reflect a sense in which one might say that 'mind extends beyond the skin', i.e. a sense in which 'mind' is a term that can be predicated of groups as well as of the individual. His assumptions also highlight the fact that notions such as 'dialogue', 'interactional dominance' (Linell, this volume, Chapter 7) and 'conversation' (Luckmann, this volume, Chapter 2) have essential implications for analysing mental functioning on the interpsychological *and* intrapsychological planes.

The general genetic law of cultural development underlies many of the best known constructs in Vygotsky's approach. For example, his notion of the 'zone of proximal development' (Vygotsky, 1978, 1987; Rogoff and Wertsch, 1984) is a particular instantiation of his more general concern with the transition from interpsychological to intrapsychological functioning, and his account of internalization (Wertsch and Stone, 1985) derives directly from it.

Mediation by signs

Vygotsky's primary emphasis in elaborating the third theme that runs throughout his writings was on the mediation provided by 'psychological tools', or signs. For this reason, I shall focus here on what may be termed semiotic mediation rather than on the broader category that covers mediation by technical tools as well. As I have argued elsewhere (Wertsch, 1985b), Vygotsky's concern with semiotic mediation is analytically prior to the other two themes in the sense that the formulation of each of these other two is grounded in some way in this one. In the case of his genetic method, this is manifested in the fact that genetic transitions are defined by the appearance of new forms of mediation or the transformation of existing ones. In the case of the social origins of individual mental functioning, it is manifested in the fact that relevant forms of interpsychological and intrapsychological functioning, as well as their interrelationships, are defined in terms of the mediational means involved. For example, his very definition of interpsychological functioning, and the transformations he saw it undergoing to form intrapsychological functioning, are grounded in semiotic criteria.

In a sense the analytic priority given to semiotic mediation in Vygotsky's writings reflects the progression of his intellectual biography. Before he began his official career as a psychologist, he spent several years reading and writing about issues of literary analysis, philology and the philosophy of language. Indeed, it was this preparation that made it possible for him to make his unique contributions to the study of human mental functioning.

Another way of making this point is to speculate on what the first two themes in Vygotsky's approach would have meant if they had not been grounded in the theme of semiotic mediation. When taken in isolation, neither of them provides many insights that were not already available in the writings of others (e.g. Baldwin, Piaget, Werner). By invoking the notion of semiotic mediation, however, Vygotsky managed to provide a novel and productive interpretation of these two themes and to extend theoretical and empirical research in a variety of other ways as well. In the end, therefore, the key to Vygotsky's original insights is to be found in the ways in which the three themes of his thought are interdefined.

The theme of semiotic mediation came to play an increasingly important role in Vygotsky's approach during the final years of his life. By 1932 he went so far as to note that semiotic analysis ('*semicheskii analiz*') is 'the only adequate method for analysing human consciousness' (Vygotsky, 1977, p. 94). Minick (1987) has documented this increasing tendency to incorporate semiotic analyses into Vygotsky's account of mental functioning as part of the 'third stage' of Vygotsky's intellectual career.

Vygotsky's approach to semiotic mediation led him to a formulation of higher mental functioning in which agency accrues to humans (either individually or in groups) *acting with mediational means*. In such an approach, agency cannot be understood by analysing either the individual or mediational means in isolation. Instead, the agent of action is the system created by the two means acting together as an irreducible whole. Among other things, this rules out the idea that mediational means simply facilitate forms of action that could occur in their absence. Instead of viewing mediational means as being somehow secondary or ancillary to an already existing form of action, Vygotsky argued that:

> by being included in the process of behavior, the psychological tool alters the entire flow and structure of mental functions. It does this by determining the structure of a new instrumental act, just as a technical tool alters the process of a natural adaptation by determining the form of labor operations. (Vygotsky, 1981b, p. 137)

As in the case of the general genetic law of cultural development, Vygotsky's view of mediational means is grounded in assumptions that challenge some of the individualistic biases permeating contemporary psychology. It suggests that just as mind extends beyond the skin in the form of interpsychological functioning, so does agency involve mediational means as well as individuals.

The specific semiotic mechanisms that Vygotsky envisioned can be summarized in terms of two basic 'potentials' (Wertsch, 1985b) that he saw in human language. On the one hand, he saw the potential for language to serve in a highly contextualized way. During early phases of ontogenesis this involves ways in which language is tied to the extralinguistic context (*ibid.*); later, speech comes to serve as its own context (a linguistic context), giving rise to phenomena such as abbreviation that characterize the structure of egocentric and inner speech. On the other hand, Vygotsky recognized the potential for language to function in decontextualized ways. In particular, his analysis of the emergence of scientific concepts is connected with the 'decontextualization of mediational means' (*ibid.*). Such decontextualization involves the process whereby linguistic expressions are lifted out of a context of communication and used as objects of reflection and analysis. Examples of this can be found in the practice of giving dictionary definitions of words. In this practice a definition is assumed to remain constant across communicative contexts. The practice of reflecting on decontextualized mediational means is specifically the kind of phenomenon that concerned Vygotsky in his account of genuine and scientific concepts.

These two general semiotic potentials are inherently tied to the other two themes that run throughout Vygotsky's writings. The highly contextualized potential is tied to the developmental processes involved in the transition from social speech (a form of interpsychological functioning) to egocentric and inner speech (forms of intrapsychological functioning). In contrast, the move towards decontextualization underlay his genetic analysis of 'complexes', 'pseudoconcepts' and 'concepts'.

It is in connection with concept development that Vygotsky made some of his most significant strides in addressing socio-cultural issues during the last years of his life. These strides are reflected in the difference between Chapters 5 and 6 of *Thinking and Speech* (Vygotsky, 1987)[1]. Chapter 5, 'An experimental study of concept development', was probably written sometime in the early 1930s. In it Vygotsky reported on research he had conducted with Sakharov (1930) in the late 1920s. Chapter 6, 'The development of scientific concepts in childhood', was written specifically for the volume *Thinking and Speech*, which was first published in 1934. Although both chapters are concerned with concept development, there is a major difference between them with respect to how this development is thought to take place. Chapter 5 deals with concept development in terms of individual mental functioning as measured in a clinical–experimental setting. Results from the Vygotsky–Sakharov block sorting task were used to document the nature of various sorts of complexes and the transition to pseudoconceptual and conceptual levels of functioning. In Chapter 6, the concern with concept development continues to occupy centre stage, but there is an important shift to considering concept development in terms of how it is tied to forms of discourse in a specific institutional context, namely, formal schooling. This shift is reflected in the terminology Vygotsky employed. In constrast to Chapter 5, where the talk is of complexes, pseudoconcepts, genuine concepts and other constructs that apply to individual mental functioning, Chapter 6 deals with 'scientific concepts', a term not employed previously. It is important to note that the Russian term involved here (*'nauchnyi'*) can be translated as 'academic' or 'scholarly' instead of 'scientific' (indeed, 'scholarly' has been used in the translation of Luria, 1976). This shift in Vygotsky's

---

1. This 1987 volume is the first complete English translation of a work by Vygotsky originally published in 1934. Two other, much abridged, translations of this 1934 volume have been published as *Thought and Language* by MIT Press in 1962 and 1986.

terminology reflects his growing concern with how specific forms of speaking and thinking are related to the socio-cultural context of the classroom. His focus had expanded beyond both intrapsychological functioning and interpsychological functioning construed in a narrow way; in place of searching for the social origins of individual mental functioning in dyads or small groups, he was concerned with how such groups are situated in a broader socio-cultural context.

This difference between Chapters 5 and 6 of *Thinking and Speech* reflects the growing interest Vygotsky had near the end of his life in the socio-cultural situatedness of mental functioning. However, it was only a beginning. For the most part, his theme about the social origins of individual mental functioning was still limited to considering dialogue as opposed to dialogism (Marková, this volume, Introduction). In order to expand upon Vygotsky's budding vision, it is necessary to expand on the notion of semiotic mediation. Semiotic mediation is the key to an expansion because it is this, in a Vygotskian approach, that serves to link socio-cultural setting with individual mental functioning: on the one hand, particular semiotic practices (e.g using language in literacy activities) reflect and help constitute socio-cultural settings; on the other hand, they shape the genesis of individual mental functioning (via the interpsychological plane).

Bakhtin's contribution to a socio-cultural approach

I shall extend Vygotsky's approach by introducing some ideas from a contemporary of his, M. M. Bakhtin (1981, 1984; Vološinov, 1973). Although there is no evidence that Vygotsky and Bakhtin ever met, or even that either read the other's work, their approaches are grounded in quite similar sets of underlying assumptions. Instead of producing identical approaches, however, the result was a great deal of complementarity. This is nowhere more evident than in connection with the issue of dialogicality. Vygotsky was no stranger to the category of dialogicality, but it did not play a central role in his account of the development of mental processes. Conversely, Bakhtin was not primarily interested in psychological issues, but he outlined a unique and powerful approach to dialogicality that has a wealth of implications for a psychology of socio-culturally situated mental processes.

Unlike many contemporary scholars of language, who take as their object of analysis linguistic form and meaning abstracted from actual conditions of use, Bakhtin focused his analytic efforts on the utterance, 'the *real unit* of speech communication' (Bakhtin, 1986, p. 71).

> Speech can exist in reality only in the form of concrete utterances of individual speaking people, speech subjects. Speech is always cast in the form of an utterance belonging to a particular speaking subject, and outside this form it cannot exist. (*ibid.*, p. 71)

As Clark and Holquist (1984) have noted, this focus on utterance did not mean that Bakhtin rejected the notion that there is constancy and systematicity in language or speech. Instead, according to him, it is in the utterance that constancy and systematicity enter into contact and struggle with unique, situated performance. Furthermore, the constancy and systematicity that he did see in language was not limited to the types of phenomena linguists typically examine. While readily acknowledging the need to study 'the specific object of linguistics, something arrived at through a completely legitimate and necessary abstraction from various aspects of the concrete life of the word' (Bakhtin, 1984, p. 181), Bakhtin argued for the need to create an alternative approach that would incorporate a concern with how utterances and the voices producing them are organized in their socio-cultural context. Specifically, he argued for the need to create an approach that transcends the concerns of individual existing disciplines, an approach that Clark and Holquist (1984) have termed 'translinguistics'.

Translinguistics is 'the study of those aspects in the life of the word [i.e. in speech], not yet shaped into separate and specific disciplines, that exceed – and completely legitimately – the boundaries of linguistics' (Bakhtin, 1984, p. 181). Bakhtin's comments indicate that translinguistics overlaps with the study of what today is called pragmatics or discourse, but no easy definitions can be created using such contemporary terms because of Bakhtin's grounding of translinguistics in a set of unique categories, especially voice and dialogicality.

In Bakhtin's account, the notion of utterance is inherently linked with that of voice, a term which refers to 'the speaking personality, the speaking consciousness' (Holquist and Emerson, 1981, p. 434). His notion of voice touches on issues of intonation, but it cannot be reduced to an analysis of vocal–auditory signals. Instead, it is more general, applying to written as well as spoken communication and conceived with the broader issues of a speaking subject's perspective, belief system, intention and world view in mind.

The inherent connection between voice and utterance derives from the fact that an utterance can exist only through being produced by a voice. For Bakhtin, one of the major shortcomings of linguistic, as opposed to translinguistic, analyses is that the units of analysis (e.g. words, sentences) are abstracted from voice. The resulting units then:

> belong to nobody and are addressed to nobody. Moreover, they in themselves are devoid of any kind of relation to the other's utterance, the other's word. (Bakhtin, 1986, p. 99)

In Bakhtin's approach, the issue of how an utterance belongs to a speaking voice as well as to others is a constant concern. It is part of his more general observation that 'Any utterance is a link in the chain of speech communication' (*ibid.*, p. 84), an observation that, in turn, means that 'Utterances are not indifferent to one another, and are not self-sufficient; they are aware of and mutually reflect one another' (*ibid*, p. 91). Indeed, this issue of how any utterance is inherently interrelated with others is at the core of Bakhtin's approach. It is the issue that underlies the most fundamental category in his approach: dialogicality.

Bakhtin's translinguistic analyses were grounded in the observation that 'The utterance is filled with *dialogic overtones*' (*ibid.*, p. 92). Indeed, 'Dialogic relationships . . . are the subject of metalinguistics [i.e. translinguistics]' (Bakhtin, 1981, p. 182). The basic concern with dialogicality manifests itself in a variety of ways. For example, Bakhtin's approach to understanding or comprehension is grounded in the idea that:

> when the listener perceives and understands the meaning . . . of speech he simultaneously takes an active, responsive attitude toward it. He either agrees or disagrees with it . . . augments it, applies it, prepares for its execution, and so on. . . . Any understanding of live speech, a live utterance, is inherently responsive, although the degree of this activity varies extremely. Any understanding is imbued with response and necessarily elicits it in one form or another: the listener becomes the speaker. (Bakhtin, 1986, p. 68)

For Bakhtin, dialogicality includes, but extends far beyond, the process whereby one speaker's concrete utterances come into contact with utterances of another speaking consciousness (e.g. in face-to-face dialogue or in the process of understanding outlined above). In addition to this 'primordial dialogism of discourse' involving a dialogic orientation of one speaker's utterances to 'others' utterances inside a *single* language' (Bakhtin, 1981, p. 275), he concerned himself with several other basic categories of dialogic orientation that fall under the heading of dialogism as outlined by Marková (this volume, Introduction). For example, he was concerned with the dialogic orientation among '"social languages" within a single *national* language' and a dialogic orientation among 'different national languages within the same *culture*' (Bakhtin, 1981, p. 275). In order to understand what Bakhtin had in mind when dealing with these two categories of dialogicality, one must turn to the notions of *language* that he was employing.

The first point to recognize in this connection is that by switching from speaking of utterances to speaking of languages, Bakhtin was making a switch from dealing with unique speech events (i.e. individual utterances produced by a voice in a unique speech event) to dealing with categories, or *types* of speech events (i.e. types of utterances produced by types of voices). Since 'the utterance itself is individual and unreproducible' (Vološinov, 1973, p. 199), any concern with types of speech events, as in the study of languages, may at first appear to fall outside the boundaries of translinguistics. This is not so, however, because unlike analyses that focus on linguistic objects abstracted from all aspects of the speech event, Bakhtin's account of languages clearly retained the notion of voice as well as various kinds of dialogicality among voices. Furthermore, he was concerned with the struggle between system and performance that gets played out in the utterance. The fact that utterances and voices (now considered as types) are inherently linked and that dialogicality is still at the centre of attention means that the analysis of languages falls within the realm of metalinguistics.

By a national language Bakhtin understands 'the traditional linguistic unities (English, Russian, French, etc.) with their coherent grammatical and semantic systems' (Holquist and Emerson, 1981, p. 430). In actuality, as Clark and Holquist (1984) point out, the notion of a unitary national language is an 'academic fiction' (p. 13) which papers over the effects of centrifugal forces that seek to stratify and change it. When he talked about dialogic orientation among national languages, Bakhtin had in mind the different ways in which the various languages are employed in different cultural settings. For example, one national language may be used at home, another in formal instructional settings and yet a third in religious ceremonies. His concern goes beyond this, however, because for him it is not simply a matter of distribution in use of various national languages; it is also a matter of how these languages and their uses are interrelated, or enter into dialogic interanimation (e.g. how one language may be used to provide counter-words to another). This is the kind of phenomenon often studied under the heading of 'code switching' in contemporary sociolinguistics (e.g. Gumperz, 1982). Bakhtin provided relatively little concrete detail on how national languages might enter into dialogic contact. In connection with social languages, however, he was more specific.

For Bakhtin, a social language is 'a discourse peculiar to a specific stratum of society (professional, age group, etc.) within a given social system at a given time' (Holquist and Emerson, 1981, p. 430). Throughout his writing, Bakhtin used a variety of terms to refer to social languages. For example, at some points he spoke of 'social speech types', and in many places he simply used the term 'language'. I shall employ the term 'social language' in what follows, the term 'social' serving to distinguish a social language from a national language.

A multitude of social languages typically exist within a single national language. Hence languages and social languages can, at least to some extent, vary independently of one another. As examples of social languages Bakhtin mentioned 'social dialects, characteristic group behavior, professional jargons, generic languages, languages of generations and age groups, tendentious languages, languages of the authorities of various circles and of passing fashions, languages that serve the specific sociopolitical purposes of the day' (Bakhtin, 1981, p. 262).

In Bakhtin's view, speakers always speak in social languages when producing unique utterances, and these social languages shape what their individual voices can say. This process of producing unique utterances by speaking in social languages involves a specific kind of dialogicality or multivoicedness that Bakhtin termed 'ventriloquation' (Bakhtin, 1981; Holquist, 1981), i.e. the process whereby one voice speaks *through* another voice or voice type as found in a social language.

> The word in language is half someone else's. It becomes 'one's own' only when the speaker populates it with his own intention, his own accent, when he appropriates the word, adapting it to his own semantic and expressive intention. Prior to this moment of appropriation, the word does not exist in a neutral and impersonal language (it is not, after all, out of a dictionary that the speaker gets his words!), but rather it exists in other people's mouths, in other people's concrete contexts, serving other people's intentions: it is from there that one must take the word, and make it one's own. (Bakhtin, 1981, pp. 293–4)

One type of social language that Bakhtin examined in particular detail was the 'speech genre'. In contrast to other types of social languages, such as the social languages of generations, speech genres have a restricted and identifiable form. However, as in the case of other types of social languages, speakers ventriloquate through speech genres, and are thereby shaped in what they can and will say. This is so even though speakers may be quite unaware of the process involved or even of the existence of speech genres.

> We speak only in definite speech genres, that is, all our utterances have definite and relatively stable typical *forms of construction of the whole*. Our repertoire of oral (and written) speech genres is rich. We use them confidently and skillfully *in practice*, and it is quite possible for us not even to suspect their existence *in theory*. Like Molière's Monsieur Jourdain who, when speaking in prose, had no idea that was what he was doing, we speak in diverse genres without suspecting that they exist. (Bakhtin, 1986, p. 78)

The approach to meaning inherent in these comments is one in which speakers 'rent' meaning, as Holquist (1981) puts it. He contrasts this with personalist theories of meaning such as those proposed by Vossler, according to which the speaker 'owns' meaning, and deconstructionist views, which hold that '"*No one* owns meaning": the very conception of meaning, to say nothing of persons, invoked in most traditional epistemologies, begins by illicitly assuming a presence whose end Nietzsche really was announcing when he let be known that God had died in history' (Holquist, 1981, p. 164).

A way of capturing and applying this theoretical perspective in concrete cases is to pose what I shall term 'the Bakhtinian question'. This question is: who is doing the talking? The pervasiveness of dialogicality in Bakhtin's view means that the answer will inevitably identify at least two voices. For example, in the case of parody, which was one of the phenomena of dialogicality, or multivoicedness, that interested Bakhtin, the effect derives from the fact that two voices, speaking simultaneously, are discernible. On the one hand, the speaking consciousness producing the concrete parodic utterance is obviously speaking; on the other hand, it is only by populating, or appropriating the utterance of another, that parody comes into being. Hence the phenomenon is inherently multivoiced.

But one need not turn to the special case of parody to witness the fundamental dialogicality of utterances. Because an utterance can be produced only by appropriating a social language, *all* utterances are inherently dialogic in the Bakhtinian view. An utterance can no more be produced without ventriloquating through one or more social languages than it can be produced without appropriating some national language such as Swedish or Japanese. For example, as I write this I am appropriating a kind of academic discourse, i.e. a social language, with its particular pattern of presentation, argumentation and so forth. This is a social language that is fairly clearly distinguishable from others that I invoke in other settings. If one asks the Bakhtinian question 'who is doing the talking?' as I produce this text, part of the answer obviously has to do with the voice associated with me as an individual, but there is an essential sense in which one can hear the social language as well. Like all social languages, it has a history and usage that extends far beyond me as an individual speaking consciousness.

Social languages as mediational means

Bakhtin's account of dialogicality has major implications for a socio-cultural approach to mind. Of particular importance for my purposes, it has implications for how one can extend Vygotsky's basic formulation of mental functioning so that its inherent relationship to cultural, historical and institutional settings can be recognized. The key to this is contained in the concept of social languages as mediational means.

As outlined above, Vygotsky recognized the power of mediational means, especially semiotic means, to shape interpsychological and intrapsychological functioning. However, the account of mediational means he used did not encourage him to specify how this functioning is tied to socio-cultural setting. His concern with the semiotic potential associated with decontextualization (this chapter, p. 69) certainly did little to encourage a view of semiotic action tied to socio-cultural setting, and his analysis of contextualized signification as reflected in his account of egocentric and inner speech (*ibid.*) rests on an account of context that does not extend beyond the interpsychological level.

A focus on social languages as mediational means, however, leads one in a quite different direction. By their very nature social languages are tied to a socio-cultural setting, a point that is reflected in their definition as forms of 'discourse peculiar to a specific stratum of society (professional, age group, etc.) within a given social system at a given time' (Holquist and Emerson, 1981, p. 430). Given the nature of social languages, an account of how they are appropriated as mediational means on the interpsychological and intrapsychological planes of functioning brings with it an inherent link to socio-cultural setting.

From the perspective of a genetic approach, a concern with notions such as ventriloquation and the renting of meaning introduces a specific set of concerns. Ontogenesis is viewed in terms of gaining increasing mastery in a variety of social languages. This is hinted at in Bakhtin's comment that 'To learn to speak means to learn to construct utterances' (Bakhtin, 1986, p. 78), utterances which 'Speech genres organize . . . in almost the same way as grammatical (syntactical) forms do' (*ibid*., pp. 78–9). The suggestion is that instead of grounding analyses of mediation and representation in utterances that supposedly belong to nobody, there is a need for an approach to meaning that is inherently grounded in dialogicality, i.e. dialogism and dialogue.

The kind of reorientation I am proposing is quite consistent with what Vygotsky seems to have had in mind in his final works on the nature of scientific concepts. Instead of viewing these concepts as some kind of individual psychological phenomena, he was beginning to view them as being part of a social language that reflects and creates a particular socio-cultural setting, namely formal schooling. While this is certainly not the only social language involved in a socio-cultural approach, it is one that does play an essential role in many societies today. Elsewhere, I have examined the social language of formal schooling under the heading of 'text based realities' (Wertsch, forthcoming).

The challenge of developing a socio-cultural approach of the type I have proposed involves several basic tasks. The key to all of these is the notion of a social language. The first essential step is to identify and characterize particular social languages. This is quite a problem since most analyses in linguistics, sociolinguistics, semiotics and other associated disciplines are not grounded in concepts similar to, or even compatible with, Bakhtin's account of dialogicality. To a large degree social languages remain invisible to these approaches.

In the case of the specific social languages peculiar to formal instructional settings, a starting point for identification and characterization can be found in the writings of social theorists such as Bourdieu (1984). He has noted that:

> all institutionalized learning presupposes a degree of rationalization. . . . [I]n place of practical schemes of classification, which are always partial and linked to practical contexts, it puts explicit,

standardized taxonomies, fixed once and for all in the form of synoptic schemas or dualistic typologies (e.g. 'classical'/'romantic'), which are expressly inculcated and therefore conserved in the memory as knowledge that can be reproduced in virtually identical forms by all the agents subject to its action. (*ibid.*, pp. 66–7)

As I have noted elsewhere (Wertsch and Minick, forthcoming), the social theoretic notion of rationality may indeed hold the key to understanding a great deal of what goes on in the discourse of formal instruction.

A second task that confronts those concerned with the issues I have outlined in this chapter is that of specifying precisely how social languages reflect and create particular socio-cultural settings. This is a task that requires a grounding in issues that range far beyond the boundaries that typically define the activities of psychologists, and can, therefore, be realistically confronted only with a great deal of interdisciplinary co-operation. Again, the ideas of social theorists such as Bourdieu (1977, 1984) can be quite helpful in such a venture.

A third essential step in this enterprise is to examine the processes whereby appropriating various social languages affects intrapsychological functioning. This is an issue that Minick and I have begun to map out in terms of Vygotsky's account of the 'zone of proximal development' (Vygotsky, 1978, p. 86; Wertsch and Minick, forthcoming).

The kind of enterprise I am proposing poses several major challenges. It seems to me, however, that it is worth the effort for at least two reasons. First, there are several pieces of the puzzle that are already available, at least *in potentia*. For example, ethnographers of speaking such as Bauman, Irvine, and Philips (1987) have recently outlined several characteristics of genres of speaking that are quite relevant to the approach, and there is a growing general appreciation of the need to take socio-cultural issues more seriously into account when trying to understand the socialization of cognitive processes (e.g. Ochs, 1988). The second reason for pursuing the line of inquiry I have mapped out here is simply that we may have no choice. Without an adequate account of mediation grounded in dialogicality, it may be impossible to deal with many of the issues raised by a socio-cultural approach to mind. If this is so, the analysis of dialogue and dialogism is not simply a new way to approach old problems: it fundamentally redefines the problems, and also the methods and theoretical constructs we currently have for addressing them.

References

Bakhtin, M. M. (1981), *The Dialogic Imagination: Four essays by M. M. Bakhtin*, M. Holquist (ed.), trans. C. Emerson and M. Holquist, Austin: University of Texas Press.

Bakhtin, M. M. (1984), *Problems of Dostoevsky's Poetics*, C. Emerson (ed.), trans. C. Emerson, Minneapolis: University of Minnesota Press; Manchester: Manchester University Press.

Bakhtin, M. M. (1986), *Speech Genres and Other Late Essays*, C. Emerson and M. Holquist (eds), trans. V. W. McGee, Austin: University of Texas Press.

Bauman, R., Irvine, J. T. and Philips, S. (1987), 'Performance, speech community, and genre: A critical review of concepts in the ethnography of speaking', *Working Papers and Proceedings of the Center for Psychosocial Studies*, 11.

Blonskii, P. P. (1921), *Ocherki po nauchnoi psikhologii (Essays in Scientific Psychology)*, Moscow: Gosudarstvennoe Izdatel'stvo.

Bourdieu, P. (1977), *Outline of a Theory of Practice*, trans. R. Nice, Cambridge: Cambridge University Press.

Bourdieu, P. (1984), *Distinction: A social critique of the judgement of taste*, trans. R. Nice, Cambridge, Mass.: Harvard University Press.

Clark, K. and Holquist, M. (1984), *Mikhail Bakhtin*, Cambridge, Mass.: Harvard University Press.

Davydov, V. V. and Radzikhovskii, L. A. (1985), 'L. S. Vygotsky's theory and the activity-oriented approach in psychology', in J. V. Wertsch (ed.), *Culture, Communication, and Cognition: Vygotskian perspectives*, New York: Cambridge University Press.

Gumperz, J. J. (1982), *Discourse Strategies*, Cambridge: Cambridge University Press.

Holquist, M. (1981), 'The politics of representation', in S. Greenblatt (ed.), *Allegory in Representation: Selected papers from the English Institute*, Baltimore: Johns Hopkins University Press.

Holquist, M. and Emerson, C. (1981), Glossary for M. M. Bakhtin, *The Dialogic Imagination*.

Hutchins, E. (forthc.), 'The social organization of distributed cognition'. Chapter to appear in a volume from the conference Socially Shared Cognition, Learning Research and Development Center, University of Pittsburgh, February, 1989.

Köhler, W. (1927), *The Mentality of Apes*, trans. from the 2nd edn by E. Winter, London: Kegan Paul.

Luria, A. R. (1971), 'Towards the problem of the historical nature of psychological processes', *International Journal of Psychology*, 6(4), 259–72.

Luria, A. R. (1976), *Cognitive Development: Its cultural and social foundations*, M. Cole and S. Cole (eds), Cambridge, Mass.: Harvard University Press.

Luria, A. R. (1981), *Language and Cognition*, J. V. Wertsch (ed.), New York: Wiley Intersciences.

Mecacci, L. (1979), *Brain and History: The relationship between neurophysiology and psychology in Soviet research*, New York: Brunner/Mazel.

Middleton, D. (1987), 'Some issues and approaches', *The Quarterly Newsletter of Comparative Human Cognition*, (special issue devoted to Collective Memory and Remembering), vol. 9(1).

Minick, N. (1987), Introduction to Vygotsky, L. S. (1987), *Thinking and Speech*, N. Minick (ed.), trans. N. Minick, New York: Plenum.
Ochs, E. (1988), *Culture and Language Development: Language acquisition and language socialization in a Samoan village*, Cambridge: Cambridge University Press.
Rogoff, B. and Wertsch, J. V. (eds) (1984), *Children's Learning in the 'Zone of Proximal Development'*, no. 23 in *New Directions for Child Development*, San Francisco: Jossey-Bass.
Sakharov, L. S. (1930), 'O metodakh issledovaniya ponyatii' (Methods for the Investigation of Concepts'), *Psikhologiya*, 3(1).
Smirnov, A. N. (1975), *Razvitie i sovremennoe sostoyanie psikhologicheskoi nauki v SSSR (The Development and Current State of Psychology in the USSR)*, Moscow: Izdatel'stvo Pedagogika.
Vološinov, V. N. (1973), *Marxism and the Philosophy of Language*, trans. L. Matejka and I. R. Titunik, New York: Seminar Press.
Vygotsky, L. S. (1934), *Myshlenie i rech': Psikhologicheskie issledovaniya (Thinking and Speech: Psychological investigations)*, Moscow and Leningrad: Gosudarstvennoe Sotsial'no-Ekonomicheskoe Izdatel'stvo.
Vygotsky, L. S. (1977), 'Iz tet'ryadei L. S. Vygotskogo' (From the notebooks of L. S. Vygotsky), *Vestnik Moskovskogo Universiteta: Seriya psikhologii* (Moscow University Record: Psychology series), 15, 89–95.
Vygotsky, L. S. (1978), *Mind in Society: The development of higher psychological processes*, M. Cole, V. John-Steiner, S. Scribner and E. Souberman (eds), Cambridge, Mass.: Harvard University Press.
Vygotsky, L. S. (1979), 'Consciousness as a problem in the psychology of behavior', *Soviet Psychology*, 17(4), 3–35.
Vygotsky, L. S. (1981a), 'The genesis of higher mental functions', in J. V. Wertsch (ed.), *The Concept of Activity in Soviet Psychology*, Armonk, N.Y.: M. E. Sharpe.
Vygotsky, L. S. (1981b), 'The instrumental method in psychology', in J. V. Wertsch (ed.), *The Concept of Activity in Soviet Psychology*, Armonk, N.Y.: M. E. Sharpe.
Vygotsky, L. S. (1987), *Thinking and Speech*, N. Minick (ed.), trans. N. Minick, New York: Plenum.
Wertsch, J. V. (ed.) (1985a), *Culture, Communication, and Cognition: Vygotskian perspectives*, New York: Cambridge University Press.
Wertsch, J. V. (1985b), *Vygotsky and the Social Formation of Mind*, Cambridge, Mass.: Harvard University Press.
Wertsch, J. V. (forthc.), 'Sociocultural setting and the zone of proximal development: The problem of text-based realities', in S. Strauss (ed.), *Culture, Schooling and Psychological Development*, New York: Ablex.
Wertsch, J. V. and Minick, N. (forthc.), 'Negotiating sense in the zone of proximal development', in M. Schwebel, C. A. Haher and N. S. Fagley (eds.), *Promoting Cognitive Growth over the Life Span*, Hillsdale, N.J.: Erlbaum.
Wertsch, J. V. and Stone, C. A. (1985), 'The concept of internalization in Vygotsky's account of the genesis of higher mental functions', in J. V. Wertsch (ed.), *Culture, Communication, and Cognition: Vygotskian perspectives*, Cambridge: Cambridge University Press.
Wertsch, J. V. and Youniss, J. (1987), 'Contextualizing the investigator: The case of developmental psychology', *Human Development*, 30, 18–31.

Zinchenko, V. P. and Gordon, V. M. (1981), 'Methodological problems in the psychological analysis of activity', in J. V. Wertsch (ed.), *The Concept of Activity in Soviet Psychology*, Armonk, N.Y.: M. E. Sharpe.

Zinchenko, V. P. and Smirnov, S. D. (1983) *Metodologicheskie voprosy psikhologii (Methodological Problems of Psychology)*, Moscow: Moscow University Press.

4 | On axiomatic features of a dialogical approach to language and mind

Ragnar Rommetveit
Department of Psychology, University of Oslo

Dialogical and monological approaches to cognition and communication

The aim of this chapter is to try to identify a core of preconceptions which may be said to define a consistently dialogical approach to human cognition and communication. My choice of terms, 'axiomatic features' and 'preconceptions' rather than 'axioms', is deliberate and based on the assumption that as *participants* in ordinary language as a 'form of life', we are imprisoned within human meaning, yet as *researchers* we are capable of reflecting upon and exploring our very embeddedness. *Understanding*, in social scientific studies, is logically prior to *explanation*. Any conceptual framework for the study of language and mind is hence bound to contain residuals about which we have to admit, with Wittgenstein (1962, p. 739), that 'there is no such thing as an interpretation of that'.

This predicament does not, in my view, imply imprisonment within a repertoire of hermeneutic methods of the kind developed and defined within the humanities. There is today an increasing concern with the subject-to-subject relation between investigator and informant across a wide range of disciplines dealing with human cognition and communication. Discontent with monological models and pleas for paradigmatic change are currently voiced by social scientists engaged in experimental research and by representatives of cognitive science (see Rommetveit, 1987, 1988a). The target of joint attacks is the preconception of the individual human mind as a mirror of an external reality. Current critiques of mainstream cognitive psychology and cognitive science may hence, from an epistemological point of view, be interpreted as a manifestation of a general 'anti-Cartesian revolution' (Rorty, 1980; Markovà, 1982).

The issue of monologically versus dialogically based studies of human cognition and communication, however, is not simply a matter of choice between alternative, fully and explicitly elaborated philosophical foundations. Nor is it merely a matter of choice between competing sets of explanatory models on the part of scholars seeking answers to identical problems within well-defined fields of empirical research. It has, rather, to do with different webs of only partially acknowledged presuppositions which – while rooted in pre-scientific notions and concerns – shape our ways of wondering about language and mind, and pervade conceptualization and problem formulation in particular ways. The ways of wondering which distinguish a consistently dialogical approach to language and mind, I shall venture to assume, are in important respects very similar across a wide range of social, scientific and humanistic disciplines. The task I have set myself is thus to bring into the open significant yet only partially acknowledged axiomatic features of a general dialogical paradigm.

A very important part of the web of presuppositions underlying a dialogical approach can be converted into statements about the social nature of humankind and the embeddedness of the individual human mind in the cultural collectivity. Wondering about such intricate issues is indeed a recurrent trade in philosophical and scientific enquiries into the human condition. Spinoza conceived of human identity as thoroughly *relational*, and this is expressed in a particularly significant way by Naess (1975, p. 46) in his interpretation of Spinoza's ethics: 'Man exists *in* personal relations as a changing centre of interactions in a field of relations.'

G. H. Mead, moreover, warned Cartesian psychologists more than half a century ago against the mistake 'that all we can call thought can be located in the organism or can be put inside the head' (Mead, 1934, p. 114). Mead maintained that the individual mind is socially constituted and its field or locus is co-extensive with its 'social activity or apparatus of social relations' (*ibid.*, p. 223). An equally articulate faith in irreducibly interactional and collective features of meaning and mind pervades the works of Gregory Bateson: two or more persons engaged in interaction constitute 'a thinking-and-acting-system' whose mental characteristics '*are immanent not in some part, but in the system as a whole*' (Bateson, 1973, p. 287).

In Mead's theory of the social origin of the self, the embeddedness of the mature individual mind in a collectivity is portrayed as a product of symbolic interaction and is thus of dialogical origin. This is also a basic and firmly shared presupposition in some of the most influential writings from the golden era of Soviet semiotics and psychology of language and thought. It is interesting that Vološinov, in his *Marxism and the Philosophy of Language* (1929/1986), and Vygotsky, in his *Thought and Language* (1934/1986), quote the same passage from Dostoevsky's *Diary of a Writer* (1873–81/1949), a passage both of them most likely had encountered in Lev Yakubinsky's (1923/1986) comprehensive study *On Dialogical Speech*, published in 1923.

The fact that Vološinov and Vygotsky did not refer to one another at all in their works is perhaps best explained by the (dialogical) truism about human discourse that what is firmly taken for granted need be neither said nor written. Their ideas were developed within an intellectual climate in which the social nature of humankind was hardly questioned at all; irreducibly collective features of individual human consciousness were acknowledged by Vološinov, Vygotsky and Bakhtin to be reflections of its dialogical nature. Thus Vološinov (1986, p. 86) conceives of the word as 'a two-sided act . . . determined equally by *whose* word it is and *for whom* it is meant'. He maintains that:

> Consciousness becomes consciousness only once it has been filled with ideological (semiotic) content, consequently, only in the process of social interaction.
>
> Individual consciousness is . . . only a tenant lodging in the social edifice of ideological signs. (*ibid.*, pp. 10, 13)

Ideas emerge, according to Bakhtin (1973), when 'voices and consciousnesses' come into contact. Even the innermost thoughts of Raskolnikov and other characters of Dostoevsky are, in Bakhtin's view, dialogical. Not yet verbalized experiences are made sense of and – to use Gadamer's (1975) expression – 'brought into language' by one mind addressing another in an attempt to, e.g. blame or justify him- or herself. A characteristic feature of such socially embedded mental activity, moreover, is *'the loophole of consciousness and the word'*, i.e. 'the retention for oneself of the possibility for altering the ultimate, final meaning of one's own words' (Bakhtin, 1984, p. 313). However:

> The life of a word is contained in its transfer from one mouth to another, from one social collective to another, from one generation to another generation. In this process the word does not forget its own path and cannot completely free itself from the power of these concrete contexts into which it has entered. (*ibid.*, p. 270)

Culture and consciousness were also major subjects of enquiry for Vygotsky, as Kozulin maintains in his Introduction to the recent English edition of *Thought and Language* (1986). Vygotsky wanted to establish psychology as a semiotic science, i.e. as the systematic investigation of human consciousness as socially constituted and embedded in a cultural collectivity. His account of the origin of egocentric speech and its transformation into inner speech is, as Wertsch (1979; this volume, Chapter 3) maintains, essentially a story about 'higher psychological processes' emerging out of social interaction. 'Thought development', Vygotsky claims, 'is determined by language, i.e., by the sociocultural experience of the child' (Vygotsky, 1986, p. 94). Later in the same work he adds: 'Thought is not merely expressed in words; it comes into existence through them' (*ibid.*, p. 128).

Such claims seem to entail epistemological presuppositions which are formulated, perhaps most explicitly and cogently, by Gadamer in his major work *Wahrheit und Methode* (1975): we get to know the world only in the sense and to the extent that it is 'brought into language'. All the contributions to a dialogical approach that I have mentioned thus far seem indeed to converge in the following aspiration: that of taking the embeddedness and situatedness of human cognition and communication for granted, while at the same time bringing those very issues into focus in theoretical analysis and scientific research. Such a dual aspiration, in my view, also pervades the current search for constructive alternatives to Cartesian models of language and mind on the part of innovators within formal semantics such as Barwise and Perry (1983), and critics of mainstream cognitive science such as Dreyfus (1979) and Winograd and Flores (1986).

Current attempts at computer simulation of human cognition and communication may thus, as suggested by Winograd (1985), be interpreted as scientific–technological extensions of an analytic–rationalist philosophical tradition concerned with formal features of pure, decontextualized human reason. In previous attempts at outlining the characteristic features of a hermeneutic–dialogical approach (Rommetveit, 1987, 1988a), I have tried to show how representational–computational models of language and mind advocated by leading representatives of mainstream cognitive science fail to capture essential features of ordinary conversation within our pluralistic world. The hero in these attempts of mine is Mr Smith, a character initially introduced by Herbert Menzel (1979) in his essay 'Meaning – who needs it?'. In my expanded versions of Menzel's mystery story, Mr Smith is a fireman from Scarsdale who, simply by mowing his lawn early one Saturday morning, helps me to demonstrate how the embeddedness of meaning and mind in a polyphonic cultural collectivity – so brilliantly illustrated by Bakhtin in his literary analysis – also pervades profane, everyday discourse.

What is going on in Mr Smith's garden, it turns out, may under different dialogically established background conditions be made sense of in a variety of different ways and be brought into language by expressions such as 'beautify the garden', 'engage in physical exercise', 'work', 'engage in leisure-time activity', and 'not work'. What is meant and understood by an expression such as 'engage in physical exercise' (and more succinctly, perhaps, in the Norwegian intransitive verb *trimme*) may, in the terminology of Barwise and Perry (1983), be described as 'a uniformity across situations' such as pushing a lawn-mower, jogging, riding an exercise-bike, etc. Moreover, the pertinent uniformity across situations can, in this case, be intersubjectively attended to only against an opaque yet essentially shared historical–cultural background of affluence, white collar work, worry about heart disease and concern with slimness and health.

My primary reason for returning to the beloved Mr Smith on this occasion is a suspicion that he may also provoke us to explore significant *formal*, axiomatic features of a consistently dialogical approach. His mowing of the lawn can be made sense of and talked about in a variety of distinctively different ways under different dialogically established background conditions. But this is also the case with any not yet verbalized state of affairs. Perspectival relativity, I shall claim, is an inherent characteristic of human cognition and part and parcel of its situatedness. This implies, in metaphorical yet pertinently spatial terms, that the very identity of any given state of affairs is contingent upon the position from which it is viewed.

Co-genetic logic

By adopting a consistently dialogical paradigm we may be forced to abandon – according to Barwise (1985, p. 21) perhaps even within formal semantics – some widely shared, yet over-optimistic presuppositions concerning the range of applicability of powerful analytic tools such as classical set theory and Boolean logic. This is the position adopted by David Herbst in recent work on alternative analytic tools (Herbst, 1987a, 1987b). In order to understand and systematically explore the world contextually rather than in modular form or as an aggregate of disconnected elements, Herbst maintains that we need a 'contextual' and 'co-genetic' logic. The foundation for the development of such a logic has been laid by Spencer-Brown in his *Laws of Form* (1969).

Spencer-Brown's point of departure is 'the primary distinction' or basic initial step in an individuation of the world into meaningful entities and aspects, i.e. the cognitive act of organizing an entirely unstructured domain into a region bounded by an otherwise entirely unknown 'outside'. The minimal unit generated by such an act is, both in Spencer-Brown's logic and Herbst's further elaboration and modification of it, a triad of elements: the *object*, its *outside* and the *boundary* between them. These elements are undefined and undefinable individually, yet mutually definable in terms of one another. Two of them – the object and its outside – strongly resemble the *figure* and *ground* of classical *Gestalt* theory of perception. Herbst has referred to neither *Gestalt* psychology nor the hermeneutic philosophers in his works on co-genetic logic thus far. However, in his formal analysis, *Gestalt* principles are clearly superordinate rather than supplementary and auxiliary epistemological assumptions. In Gadamer's view, this is a unique and distinctive formal feature of a genuinely hermeneutic approach (see Gadamer, 1975, p. 455).

Herbst (1987a, 1987b) and Rasmussen (1986) elaborate and transform Spencer-Brownian logic into process networks having the characteristics of contextual systems, i.e. systems which 'do not normally permit decomposition into component elements without loss or transformation of their characteristics' (Herbst, 1987a, p. 2). Let us now examine the co-genetic logic currently under construction by Herbst and his co-workers as a potential tool for formulating in a more stringent and axiomatic fashion important presuppositions inherent in a dialogical approach. Consider, for instance, the web of presuppositions concerning the perspectival relativity of human cognition and organism–environment interaction in general.

Marková, discussing such issues in terms of Hegelian logic of interaction of opposites, seems to capture the gist of dialogical presuppositions within this realm in the general claim that 'the organism and its environment emerge together' (Marková, 1987, p. 288). This is precisely what is assumed by Herbst about the relationship between agent and object in his extended formal analysis of the canonical act of cognition. As indicated above, the object is first described as merely making a primary distinction. Nothing is said about the agent at this stage. It is the object, its outside and the boundary between them that constitute the emerging structure. In a further elaboration of this structure, Herbst claims that the *agent* (*qua* 'cognizing' agency) comes into being in the primary cognitive act, and (subjective) *time* is introduced in terms of the *before* and *after* arising in the making of the distinction. He maintains that 'the primary distinction can represent the producer, who constitutes himself as a bounded region in the making of a distinction, or it can represent the object' (Herbst, 1987a, p. 3). Agent and object of cognition are thus individually undefinable. They can only be defined mutually, in terms of one another.

Herbst (*ibid.*) explores the duality of the Observer and the Observed as mutually interdependent entities in simple cases of cognition of spatial relations, and formal features of the duality are portrayed as specific patterns within process networks. A true statement such as 'object A is to the left of object B' is thus informative either of the spatial location of the two objects or of the position from which they are viewed, depending upon whether the viewer's position or the location of the objects is already known. This simple observation may serve to bring into the open the fate of truth-conditional semantics within a dialogical paradigm if we acknowledge the perspectival relativity of human cognition as part of its kernel of presuppositions: in order to decide whether what is asserted about any particular state of affairs is true, we must in principle first identify the position from which it is viewed and brought into language.

A position may be fixed, universally shared and hence in some sense intersubjectively identified, and yet be unknown precisely because it is universally shared. Pervasive and firmly shared background conditions of human cognition due to biological and ecological constants, as a rule, remain inaccessible to reflective consciousness and entirely unacknowledged as long as they stay fixed. Such conditions endow human discourse with naïve confidence in 'an intersubjective world, common to all of us' (Schutz, 1945, p. 534). In conjunction with firmly shared cultural background conditions they constitute basic prerequisites for a linguistically mediated convergence of attention, e.g. for convergence of attention on to objects and events mediated by expressions such as 'lawn' and 'mowing the lawn' in everyday conversations about gardening in Scarsdale.

Identification of the position from which a given state of affairs is viewed, as a prerequisite for identifying that state of affairs, is of no practical relevance under conditions which offer us no options at all with respect to perspectives. Empirical evidence, however, such as observations of convergence of attention onto lawns mediated by the word 'lawn', by no means undermines the assumption of the cogenesis of the Observer and the Observed in co-genetic logic. This assumption does not prohibit intersubjectively attended to objects in our *Lebenswelt*, but provokes us to ponder our own contribution to the constitution of such objects.

In order to ponder that contribution seriously and *on experiential grounds* we would have to transcend the human condition in miraculous ways and, for instance, for a while borrow the sensory equipment and general biologically determined potentials and constraints of organisms such as frogs and butterflies. Transcendence of pervasive ecological background conditions can in principle, however, be achieved by technological exploitation of natural scientific knowledge. In order to learn by experience how the meaning of 'on' in simple everyday expressions such as 'the cat is on the mat' is contingent upon our location within a gravitational field we can, today, leave the earth, spread out differently arranged dyads of cat-in-spatial-contact-with-mat around us, and engage in conversation about them while ourselves floating about in outer space (Searle, 1978).

Perspectival relativity

On the decontextualization of dialogically based 'ordinary' language

Such excursions into transcendental philosophy and outer space make us realize that the issue of the embeddedness of the individual human mind in a cultural collectivity is itself embedded within a far more inclusive web of problems concerning background conditions. In view of these more inclusive and general background conditions of human cognition, what, more precisely is implied by the presupposition of its inherent perspectival relativity? Is the notion that cognition is entirely devoid of relativity merely a misleading Utopian idea or is it, on the contrary, not only attainable but already attained and indeed a distinctive feature of the kind of advanced scientific knowledge which helped us reach outer space? How can knowledge presumed devoid of perspectival relativity be distinguished from the inherently perspectival cognition of states of affairs devoid of reflexive access to the position from which they are viewed?

A hypothetical organism entirely without options with respect to perspectives would, I imagine, inhabit a monistic world which could in principle be exhaustively explored and described without any recourse to co-genetic, contextual logic. The identity operation of Boolean logic and classical set theory is unconditionally valid in the individuation of such a world into components, and truth-conditional semantics could hence be employed without constraints. The resultant exhaustive scientific description would mirror in a perfect fashion that peculiar organism's entire *Lebenswelt*. From within, it would be entirely devoid of perspectival relativity, yet from the reflective scientific observer's point of view it would be merely a fragment of the 'real' world, viewed from one particular and firmly fixed position.

At first glance, enclaves of scientifically established knowledge within highly advanced and specialized domains display a striking resemblance to our hypothetical mini-world. Such enclaves are not inhabited by our strange and fictitious organism though, and for that reason they are unintelligible from within. Scientific insight into a domain is established, not through dialogues with organisms inhabiting it, but very often with the aid of technology transcending our human sensory equipment. What is brought into language in any given advanced scientific text is thus not simply one particular fragment of our holistic, multifaceted and immediately meaningful *Lebenswelt*, but a systematically disambiguated and transformed version of such a fragment.

Werner Heisenberg, the eminent physicist, challenges us to search for the foundation of even the most advanced kind of scientific knowledge in our intersubjectively meaningful world.

> We know that any understanding must be based finally upon natural language because it is only there we can be certain to touch reality. (Heisenberg, 1965, p. 211)

What kind of a bridge between ordinary language and advanced scientific texts has Heisenberg in mind when making such a general claim? How, more specifically, does our contextual and perspectival understanding of the world relate to scientific fragments of it in a modular form or as aggregates of atomic 'facts'?

In order to pursue these issues I shall adopt a historical stance and, very briefly, explore instances of the ramification of ordinary language into scientific, technological and other highly specialized professional terminologies. Consider, for instance, the verb 'work' as it is spontaneously used in conversations about Mr Smith by people concerned with, e.g. his alleged laziness or availability to go fishing (Rommetveit, 1987). Descendants of that verb are today encountered in a number of different fields of scientific enquiry such as ergometrics, ergonomics, etc. Precision in scientific terms, however, is gained at the cost of perspectival relativity. The emancipation of a term from its origin in everyday language may, indeed, for want of better indices, serve as a fairly reliable measure of its scientific status.

Just as fathers have offspring, so too does the vernacular word 'father'. What is striking in a survey of the word's offspring across different scientific and specialized professional terminologies, is the distinctive differences, rather than any resemblances between siblings. The descendant of 'father' within genetics, for instance, is necessarily stripped of most of the meaning potential it has in everyday use. Aspects of fatherhood foregrounded within other domains of scientific and professional expertise such as the sociology of kinship roles and laws about inheritance of property are invisible from the stance adopted by the scientific geneticist and evade his or her structuring of 'reality' into elements and modules.

States of affairs studied inside various enclaves of scientific and professional expertise provide unequivocal and *different* truth conditions on the use of words such as 'work' and 'father', because the states of affairs dealt with inside any given such enclave are viewed from one particular and firmly fixed position. Everyday use of the words, on the other hand, is pervaded by polysemy and perspectival relativity. Mr Smith's activity in his garden, for example, is viewed and brought into language as 'work' by two women chatting about his alleged laziness, yet as 'not work' by one of these women shortly afterwards in a conversation with one of Mr Smith's friends who wonders whether he is free to go fishing. Consider, furthermore, the word 'father' in a lay dispute between two men, each of whom claims that he is the 'real' father of a particular child: one of the men may be the child's father *by blood*, the other by virtue of already established *reciprocal roles*. Notice, finally, how an expression such as 'inherit' is spontaneously and meaningfully used in everyday discourse about both human traits and money.

Fixation of perspectives

Ramification of ordinary human language into scientific terminologies is, in view of the random illustrations given above, clearly an irreversible process. Scientific knowledge of fragments of the world in a modular form or as aggregates of disconnected elements is developed out of a holistic, contextual and inherently perspectival understanding, i.e. by compartmentalization of our *Lebenswelt* into different domains of scientific knowledge and by fixation of perspective within such separated and closed domains. This is very likely what Heisenberg has in mind when he claims that natural language constitutes the ultimate foundation of any understanding and our only firm contact with reality. As Herbst (1987a) and Rasmussen

(1986) show, all of Boolean logic can be derived from co-genetic logic (by fixation of 'context'), but this is not so vice versa.

Perspective fixations due to emerging and increasingly shared cultural background conditions and concerns imply *reality fixations (Wirklichkeitsfestlegungen)*. Such reality fixation – usually of a normative nature – is of particular significance in action-oriented knowledge (Luckmann, 1988, p. 200). As Barwise maintains, 'anything humans systematically use is an invariant across situations so that they can step back and objectify it, and so treat it as a thing in its own right' (Barwise, 1985, p. 3). Consider, for instance, that aspect of Mr Smith's behaviour in his garden which is brought into language by the Norwegian verb *trimme*. Imagine the following episode (see Rommetveit, 1987, p. 86). A married couple is driving by. The moment they catch sight of Mr Smith, the wife points her finger, first at her husband's protruding belly and then at the slim figure behind the lawn-mower, saying 'That's what you ought to do!'. Notice that the referent of 'That' in such a case is hardly captured by an expression such as 'mowing the lawn'. What is meant by the wife in the car is not at all that her obese husband should replace Mr Smith and start mowing his lawn. Nor is it necessarily a reminder that their own lawn ought to be mowed. Indeed, the couple may very well live in a flat and have no lawn of their own at all. The 'thing' onto which their attention converges is, I shall argue, a convergence onto a socially constructed and fixated reality, an invariant across situations which was neither 'seen' by ordinary Norwegians nor brought into their language in a lexicalized form a century ago.

Wittgenstein's later philosophy of language can, as Baker and Hacker suggest, be interpreted as a crusade against 'the illusion, which has dominated European philosophy, that language has foundations in simple concepts' (Baker and Hacker, 1980, p. 163). This, I have maintained, is also the illusion pervading representational models of language and mind elaborated in terms of 'internal mental representations' of sense as Frege conceived of it (Rommetveit, 1988a). A dialogical approach, on the other hand, is unequivocally non-representational. 'Literal' meanings of everyday words such as 'work' or 'father' cannot, in view of the irreversible development of conceptual scientific knowledge from perspectival understanding, be assessed as conceptual or prototypical representational states within the individual human mind, not even if such states are supplemented by specific 'default values' mirroring pervasive background conditions (Johnson-Laird, 1987).

Such 'literal' meanings, however, constitute significant *social* realities in our highly literate societies, serving as jointly endorsed standards of correctness in everyday discourse and hence as constraints on the negotiability of meaning. The feedback upon ordinary language from its ramifications into scientific technological terminologies, when taken in conjunction with the impact of literacy and viewed within a dialogical paradigm, would constitute a most fascinating topic for diachronic studies. Such studies might help to reveal a pervasive written language bias in linguistics, unacknowledged components of normative idealization in updated and literally literal dictionary meanings of expressions, and significant (even though most likely unintended) contributions by eminent scholars such as Frege and Descartes to modern, scientifically elaborated versions of the myth of literal meaning (see Linell, 1982; Rommetveit, 1988b).

Scientific terminology appears, from within any given closed domain, to be devoid of competing human concerns and hence, in some sense, to be disinterested and value-free. Defenders of orthodox analytic–rationalist philosophical positions may accordingly invite us to view science as institutionalized 'pure' human reason. Cognition emancipated from human motives and concerns, they may argue, is accordingly more than just a notion generated by normative idealization. However, what appears as *emancipation* from human concerns from within the enclaves of scientific enquiry is, from a dialogical and co-genetic point of view, *fixation*. Fixation of the position from which states of affairs are to be viewed necessarily implies a choice among the multiple possible and fluctuating concerns which pervade our pre-scientific contextual understanding of those states of affairs.

Consider, once more, the dispute between the two men concerning which of them is the rightful father of a particular child. Let us imagine that the one who makes his claim on the basis of established role relationship rather than blood is a geneticist. In his laboratory he may even – unknowingly – have helped to establish the biological fatherhood of his opponent, yet nevertheless he argues for his own case in terms of the superordinate significance of interpersonal relations. This by no means proves that the study of genes is devoid of human concern. On the contrary: laboratory evidence may become of crucial relevance if, for instance, a dispute is brought into court. However, the fixation of concern within genetics, a 'pure' and natural science, constrains in distinctive ways its role in human decision-making within our only partially shared and contextually understood world.

This constraint may, by defenders of orthodox analytic–rationalist positions, be expressed in generalized form as a prohibition against deriving 'ought' from 'is'. By adopting a dialogical and co-genetic stance, however, we are in a position to explore the other side of the coin. States of affairs in everyday discourse are brought into language under conditions of perspectival relativity. The range of possible perspectives is accordingly, in part, a reflection of the range of possible human interests and concerns. *Signification* is necessarily imbued, therefore, with human *significance* and the investigation of meaning within ordinary language is, as Hilary Putnam (1978, p. 189) maintains, in certain significant respects a 'moral science'.

The ontogenesis of dialogicity

Implications, such as those outlined above, of the general principle of perspectival relativity, may possibly, if further elaborated, become acknowledged as additional axiomatic features of a dialogical approach. The principle as such, however, is meaningful only within an internally consistent and more inclusive axiomatic core. Let us at this stage therefore return to previously discussed and quoted 'classical' contributions to the dialogical approach and, more specifically, to claims made in those contributions about the embeddedness of the individual mind in a cultural collectivity and the inherently social-interactional features of language. These claims, we remember, seem to converge in the presupposition that the individual mind somehow and in some very important sense is dialogically constituted.

The convergence of these claims is, in my view, captured in a bold and brilliant way by Stein Bråten in recent theoretical works in which he proposes to capture the alleged dialogicity of the mind and portray it in a formally stringent and axiomatic fashion (Bråten, 1984, 1987). His point of departure is systems theory and cognitive science, and his proposed dialogical model of mind is portrayed in contrast to other types of model already available, the *representational models* offered by mainstream cognitive science, and *autopoietical models* of the kind developed by Maturana and Varela (1980). Neither of these captures the dialogical nature of mind presupposed within a consistently dialogical approach.

Bråten, on the other hand, gives the presupposition regarding the inherent dialogicity of the human mind an explicitly axiomatic form by postulating an inborn 'virtual other', i.e. by assuming that the human infant, as far as mental development is concerned, is biologically grounded as a dyadically operative and embedded entity rather than as an operationally closed monad. Dyadic embeddedness, moreover, implies dialogical closure. Thus 'By virtue of the dialogical closure involving his virtual other, the individual is able to engage in a dialogical circle with his actual other without any qualitative jump' (Bråten, 1987, p. 5).

What is implied by the postulated dyadic embeddedness and dialogical closure is illuminated in theoretical analyses of proto-conversation between infant and adult caretaker. The plausibility of Bråten's postulate is corroborated by observations from infant research interpreted as evidence for inborn 'primary intersubjectivity' (see e.g., Trevarthen and Logotheti, 1987). The presuppositions that the human mind is co-extensive with its social activity and that the word is a two-sided act may thus, it seems, be derived from a basic and plausible assumption about systemic properties of the embryonic, pre-verbal mind, properties distinctively different from those implied by representational and autopoietic models.

It therefore seems that a genuinely social dimension must be added to the canonical act of cognition of co-genetic logic: the agent comes into being in this act as a *self–other duality*. The other remains throughout the process of socialization, and language acquisition is asymmetrical as far as meaning is concerned. It is the small child rather than his or her adult caretaker (Trevarthen and Logotheti, 1987) who has to observe the listener's face and reactions in order to find out what is meant by his or her own utterance. Even under such asymmetrical conditions, though, the dialogical circle involves an 'attunement to the attunement of the other' (Barwise and Perry, 1983) on the part of both conversation partners.

The self–other duality is reflected, as was demonstrated by Bakhtin and Vološinov, in the subtle impact on the way in which some state of affairs is brought into language of 'for whom the words are meant'. Thus, in face-to-face dialogues under conditions of symmetry the duality may be described as a mirroring of a Self in another Self, and vice versa: 'The common situation includes him-for-me, and it also of course includes me-for-him' (Luckmann, 1983, p. 83). The canonical situation-of-utterance within a dialogical approach is inherently social and circular. The canonical utterance is hence not the autonomous assertion that it is assumed to be by Searle when he states his 'principle of expressibility' – a principle which has the consequence that 'non-literalness, ambiguity, and incompleteness . . . are not theoretically essential to linguistic communication' (Searle, 1969, p. 21).

Perspective setting and 'attunement to the attunement of the other'

What, then, is the canonical utterance within an axiomatically founded dialogical approach to language and mind? The answer, I shall argue, is *the answer*. Let me for the last time return to Mr Smith or, rather, to his wife. Imagine her sitting alone in the kitchen, absorbed in worries about her marital relations and the prospect of divorce. The only way she can make sense of her husband's mowing the lawn at such an early hour is by supposing that he is evading her company. This, let us assume, is also the gist of what she is mumbling to herself when suddenly the telephone rings. Her friend at the other end of the line initiates their chat by asking: 'That lazy husband of yours, is he in bed?'. Mrs Smith answers: 'No, Mr Smith is **working** this morning, he is mowing the lawn.' A short time afterwards Mrs Smith receives another call, this time from Mr Jones who, she tacitly takes it for granted, it being usually the case when he calls, wants to enquire whether Mr Smith is free to go fishing with him. He asks: 'Is your husband working?'. This time Mrs Smith answers: 'No, Mr Smith is **not working** this morning, he is mowing the lawn.' On both occasions Mrs Smith is telling the truth. The truth, however, on each separate occasion is *situated*, i.e. bound by an intersubjectively accepted perspective and a temporarily shared concern. So, I shall claim, are the potential truths of all proper answers. Even what Mrs Smith in her marital worries is mumbling to herself is meaningful – if and only if we conceive of it as an answer to some question. The question may be raised by her, yet from a position which in principle could be adopted by others.

In order to deal with the perspectivity of human cognition within a dialogical approach, therefore, it is necessary, as Graumann (1988) has shown, to transcend the 'egological' constraints inherent in Husserl's phenomenology of perspectives. *Perspective setting* in human conversation is essential for the transformation of human subjectivity into temporary states of *intersubjectivity*, i.e. of convergence of attention onto relevant aspects of the talked-about state of affairs. The 'inner horizon' of Mr Jones entails, as a prominent potentiality of further experience, the prospect of going fishing with Mr Smith that Saturday morning. This, of course, cannot *in toto* become Mrs Smith's 'inner horizon'. Her 'attunement to the attunement of the other' consists in adopting a position attuned to Mr Jones' concern, a position from which the 'leisure-time activity' rather than, e.g. the *'trimme'* aspect of her husband's mowing of the lawn acquires salience. The Observer–Observed duality is clearly revealed by the expressions 'working' and 'not working' in the two telephone conversations. What is made known about one and the same 'external' state of affairs on the two occasions is inextricably fused with different, yet in each case intersubjectively endorsed, concerns.

The choice of *the answer* as the prototypical utterance within a dialogical paradigm follows, I venture to maintain, from the assumptions of the dialogicity of mind and of the perspectival relativity inherent in ordinary language. In view of these assumptions, what is *asserted* by an utterance (i.e. its propositional content) can only be assessed relative to what is jointly presupposed by conversation partners in terms of shared background conditions and perspective. Furthermore, dyadic control of intersubjectively endorsed perspective when two partners engage in conversation about a given state of affairs is, within a dialogical paradigm, a matter of negotiation of meaning. The existence of options regarding perspectives grounded in different and even conflicting commitments and concerns raises hitherto largely unexplored problems of *distribution of epistemic responsibility*, i.e. responsibility for making sense of the talked-about state of affairs and bringing it into language.

Consider, for instance, the following plausible continuation of the chat between the two previously mentioned women. Mrs Smith's friend, having been told that Mr Smith is working – mowing the lawn – says: 'Is he really? Is he **working hard?**'. The sustained topic, we notice, is in this case determined by the interrogator's concern about Mr Smith's alleged laziness. Mrs Smith's friend was thus the one who set the perspective at the very beginning of their conversation. Her concern has become a joint concern, a *'quaestio'* (Klein and Stutterheim, 1988), being pursued by the two women in co-operation in such a way as to lend coherence to their chat as a text. It is nevertheless Mrs Smith who has brought her husband's activity in the garden into language as 'work'. Assuming that she has been properly attuned to her conversation partner, she has hence made the claim that Mr Smith is actually exerting himself and engaged in muscular effort rather than – as her sceptical friend may suspect – practising a lazy and leisurely version of lawn-mowing.

The word 'working' uttered by Mrs Smith's friend in the question above is thus echoing Mrs Smith's 'voice' (Bakhtin, 1984; Wertsch, 1988). What it meant by 'hard', moreover, is *bound* to the referent of 'working' as a temporarily shared social reality (Rommetveit, 1974, p. 90), i.e. to a *categorization* made by Mrs Smith within a *perspective* set by her friend. The latter may in fact be reluctant to accept such a categorization if, for instance, it turns out that Mr Smith's lawn-mower requires no more effort on the part of its operator than that which is necessary to drive a car. The expression 'working hard' can therefore, from a linguistic point of view, be explicated as an instance of 'construction of properties under perspectives' (Bartsch, 1987). The two women engaged in constructing a temporarily partially shared *Lebenswelt* are thus epistemically dependent upon each other and co-responsible for the ensuing product.

Analysis of dialogues 'from within'

Empirical studies of conversations within a consistently dialogical paradigm therefore require, as a minimum, a three-step analysis of *individual contributions* (Markovà, 1987, pp. 294–5, and this volume, Chapter 6; Foppa, this volume, Chapter 8). As Linell maintains: 'Topic perspectives are normally the emergent products of sequences of turns (or of long monological turns)' (Linell, this volume, p. 164). They may be heavily constrained by genre and within institutionally determined settings such as police interrogations and court trials, yet even under such conditions of asymmetry with respect to epistemic responsibility, they are no doubt dyadically and co-operatively established. In order, therefore, to capture genetic continuity across transformations and/or the progressive differentiation of a topic during any given coherent stretch of discourse, we have to examine retro- as well as pro-active linkages, i.e. *response* as well as *initiative* components of individual contributions (Linell and Gustavsson, 1987).

H. H. Clark and his associates have tried to account for the ways in which conversation partners manage to 'ground' a proposed topic of discourse, i.e. how they co-operate in such a way as to make it a shared, intersubjectively endorsed topic. They conceive of a conversation as a dyadically organized activity, proceeding contribution by contribution rather than utterance by utterance. A *contribution* is 'a stretch of talk in which the participants specify and ground the content of a coherent piece of information' (Clark and Schaefer, 1987, p. 20); *grounding* consists in placing 'the topical content . . . what the conversation is about . . . among their shared beliefs . . . technically their mutual beliefs . . .' (*ibid.*). The outcome of successful grounding is thus convergence of attention/intention on to talked-about referents, such as *The New York Times* (Clark, Shreuder and Buttrick, 1983) or *Julia* (Clark and Schaefer, 1987, p. 22).

Expressions such as 'New York Times' and 'Julia', however, are rigid designators. They designate 'the same object in all possible worlds' (Kripke, 1977, p. 78) and are entirely undetermined with respect to perspectives on the talked-about state of affairs. This type of example may tempt us to believe that we as researchers can in principle gain access to a dialogically established topic 'from the outside', without delving into intricate issues of socially negotiated perspective setting – and taking. This may also hold true for locally determined topics, for instance for *Julia* in an utterance such as 'I just saw **Julia**'. The *local quaestio* may in such a case simply be 'Julia who?' (Clark and Schaefer, 1987, p. 23), i.e. a matter of selecting one and the same unique particular among a set of entities (such as persons, pets, ships, etc.), all named 'Julia'. It is no doubt essential for two conversation partners to have one and the same Julia in mind in any meaningful dialogue about her.

Sustained external anchorage of discourse by means of a proper name or some other rigid designator does not, however, prohibit transformation or progressive differentiation of a dialogically developing topic at all. Consider, for instance, the following hypothetical conversation (see Rommetveit, 1974, pp. 45–9).

1. A: Do you know **Ingmar Bergman**?
2. B: Yes, isn't **he** wonderful? Show me some Bergman movies I have never seen, and I bet I'll be able to pick out the ones **he** has made from among any number of films you consider very similar to them.
3. A: Do you know **him** personally? **He** is supposed to arrive here any moment, and I wonder whether you could point **him** out to me.
4. B: I am sorry. I don't know what **he** looks like.

Let us assume that in this case the problems of grounding (as indeed in most cases of everyday discourse) dealt with by Clark and associates have been resolved: A and B are the whole time talking about one and the same Ingmar Bergman. All expressions in bold type are hence co-referential and anaphorically anchored in 'Ingmar Bergman' in 1. A's initial question seems to be the *quaestio*, i.e. 'the question which the text in its entirety is produced to answer' (Klein and Stutterheim, 1988, p. 5).

This *quaestio* – whether or not B knows Ingmar Bergman – entails at the beginning of the dialogue what John Shotter (1981) has aptly labelled a 'multiply determinable indeterminacy'. Knowing Ingmar Bergman may mean having some knowledge about Bergman the artist and/or having some information of potential gossip value about his private life and/or simply being able to recognize his face, etc. Which one(s) of such potential aspects is/are going to be jointly attended to is left entirely open at stage 1 of the dialogue. This leaves B – although committed to answering A's question – free to adopt the stance of an aesthete and a connoisseur of Bergman's movies, or to attribute some other qualities to him. The attribution of qualities is, as Bartsch maintains, 'determined with respect to ideals, purposes, aims and goals which people have with respect to other beings . . .' (Bartsch, 1987, p. 301). Wonderful artists may be transformed into nasty persons by conversation partners jointly engaged in prying into their private lives.

B's initiative in stage 2 is perfectly appropriate in view of A's opening question. What he considers so 'wonderful' is at least partially defined as he proceeds to specify his own position within a space of intersubjectively endorsable perspectives on the state of affairs to be talked about. He even suggests procedures by which his claim that he knows Ingmar Bergman can be empirically verified. The intersubjectively endorsed topic at the end of stage 2 is thus specified by a perspective set by B within constraints imposed by his conversation partner. A's next question, 3, confirms that he has taken B's perspective: being assured that they are talking about one and the same Ingmar Bergman and impressed by B's alleged knowledge about him as an artist, he now proceeds to inquire about a matter of immediate and practical concern.

The *quaestio*, however, is still whether B knows Ingmar Bergman. If we disregard the Observer–Observed duality inherent in human cognition and the talker–talked-about duality inherent in verbal communication, we may easily become trapped by unwarranted identity assumptions in a linguistic analysis of anaphorically connected expressions. The pronouns 'he' in B's affirmative response and exclamation of praise in (2) and 'he' in his apology for not knowing what he looks like in 4 are co-referential and anchored in the expression 'Ingmar Bergman' in 1. B's two responses, it seems, can thus be condensed into a contradiction: he knows *and* does not know Ingmar Bergman.

Such apparent contradictions disappear once we venture to assess topics of human discourse 'from within'. What attracts our attention and theoretical interest is then, as suggested above, transformation and development of dyadically established topics under conditions of negotiated and joint epistemic responsibility on the part of conversation partners.

Perspective relativity and the fluctuating understanding of our *Lebenswelt* from within are transcended, however, by the fixation of perspective within separate and separated domains such as technological, professional and scientific discourse. Indeed, much of the socialization of the individual mind seems to consist of appropriating, populating or ventriloquating through social languages. (Wertsch, this volume, Chapter 3 pp. 76–7). The story of a dialogically constituted individual mind embedded in a cultural collectivity therefore becomes, essentially, an account of the 'decontextualization of meaning in contexts of social practices' (Linell, 1989), an endorsement of collectively accepted standards of correctness of interpretation, and a commitment to historically–socially constructed shared social realities.

References

Baker, G. P. and Hacker, P. M. S. (1980) *Wittgenstein: Understanding and meaning*, Oxford: Blackwell.
Bakhtin, M. (1984)[1] *Problems of Dostoevsky's Poetics*, trans. C. Emerson, Minneapolis: University of Minnesota Press; Manchester: Manchester University Press.
Bartsch, R. (1987), 'The construction of properties under perspectives', *Journal of Semantics*, 5, 293–320.
Barwise, J. (1985), 'Situations, sets, and the axiom of foundation', Mimeo, Stanford University.
Barwise, J. and Perry, J. (1983), *Situations and Attitudes*, Cambridge, Mass.: M. I. T. Press.
Bateson, G. (1973), *Steps to an Ecology of Mind*, Suffolk: Palladin.
Bråten, S. (1984), 'The third position. Beyond artificial and autopoietic reduction', *Kybernetes*, 13, 157–63.
Bråten, S. (1987), 'Dialogical mind: The infant and the adult in proto-conversation' in M. Carvallo (ed.), *Nature, Cognition, and System*, Dordrecht: Reidel.
Clark, H. H. and Schaefer, E. (1987), 'Collaborating on contributions to conversations', *Language and Cognitive Processes*, 2' 19–41.
Clark, H. H., Shreuder, R. and Buttrick, S. (1983), 'Common ground and the understanding of demonstrative reference', *Journal of Verbal Learning and Verbal Behavior*, 22, 245–58.
Dostoevsky, F. M. (1873–81/1949), *Diary of a Writer*, trans. B. Brasol, 2 vols, New York, 1949: Scribners; New York, 1973: Octagon Books.
Dreyfus, H. L. (1979), *What Computers Can't Do. The limits of artificial intelligence*, New York: Harper.
Gadamer, H. G. (1975), *Wahrheit und Methode*, Tübingen: J. C. B. Mohr.
Graumann, C. F. (1988), 'Perspective setting and taking in verbal interaction', in R. Dietrich and C. F. Graumann (eds.), *Language Processing in Social Context*, Amsterdam: North Holland.
Heisenberg, W. (1965), 'The role of modern physics in the development of human thinking', in F. T. Severin (ed.), *Humanistic Viewpoints in Psychology*, New York: McGraw-Hill.
Herbst, D. (1987a), 'Co-genetic logics. The eight process networks', Oslo, doc. 1/87 from Work Research Institutes.

Herbst, D. (1987b), 'Man and Machine. The different nature of contextual and modular functioning', Oslo, doc. 21/87 from Work Research Institutes.
Johnson-Laird, P. N. (1987), 'The mental representation of the meaning of words', *Cognition*, 25, 189–211.
Klein, W. and Stutterheim, C. von (1988), 'Referential movement in description and narrative discourse', unpublished paper.
Kripke, S. (1977), 'Identity and necessity', in S. P. Schwartz (ed.), *Naming, Necessity and Natural Kinds*, Ithaca: Cornell University Press.
Linell, P. (1982), *The Written Language Bias in Linguistics*, Studies in Communication, 2, Linköping: Department of Communication Studies.
Linell, P. (1989), 'The embeddedness of contextualization in the contexts of social practices' forthcoming, in *Festschrift for Ragnar Rommetveit*, A. Heen Wold (ed.).
Linell, P. and Gustavsson, L. (1987), *Initiativ och respons. Om dialogens dynamik, dominans och koherens*, Studies in Communication, 15, University of Linköping.
Luckmann, T. (1983), *Life-World and Social Realities*, London: Heinemann.
Luckman, T. (1988) 'Grundformen der gesellschaft lichen Vermittlung des Wissens: Kommunikative Gattungen', *Kölner Zeitschritt für Soziologie und Sozialpsychologie*, Sonderheft 27, 191–211.
Markovà, I. (1982), *Paradigms, Thought and Language*, Chichester and New York: Wiley.
Markovà, I. (1987), 'On the interaction of opposites in psychological processes', *Journal for the Theory of Social Behaviour*, 17, 279–99.
Maturana, H. P. and Varela, F. J. (1980), *Autopoiesis and Cognition: The realization of the living*, Dordrecht: Reidel.
Mead, G. H. (1934), *Mind, Self and Society from the Standpoint of a Behaviorist*, Chicago: University of Chicago Press.
Menzel, H. (1979), 'Meaning – Who needs it?' in M. Brenner, P. Marsh and M. Brenner (eds), *The Social Context of Methods*, London: Croom-Helm.
Naess, A. (1975), *Freedom, Emotion and Self-Subsistence. The Structure of a Central Part of Spinoza's Ethics*, Oslo: Oslo University Press.
Putnam, H. (1978), *Meaning and the Moral Sciences*, London: Routledge & Kegan Paul.
Rasmussen, P. (1986), 'Short note on binary connections', Mimeo, University of Oslo.
Rommetveit, R. (1974), *On Message Structure: A framework for the study of language and communication*, London: Wiley.
Rommetveit, R. (1987), 'Meaning, context and control: Convergent trends and controversial issues in current social-scientific research on human cognition and communication', *Inquiry*, 30, 77–99.
Rommetveit, R. (1988a), 'On human beings, computers, and representational–computational versus hermeneutic–dialogical approaches to human cognition and communication', in H. Sinding-Larsen (ed.), *Artificial Intelligence and Language. Old Questions in a New Key*, Oslo: Tano.
Rommetveit, R. (1988b), 'On literacy and the myth of literal meaning', in R. Säljö (ed.), *The Written World*, Heidelberg: Springer.
Rorty, R. (1980), *Philosophy and the Mirror of Nature*, Princeton: University of Princeton Press.
Schutz, A. (1945), 'On multiple realities', *Philosophical and Phenomenological Research*, 5, 533–76.

Searle, J. R. (1969), *On Speech Acts*, Cambridge: Cambridge University Press.
Searle, J. R. (1978), 'Literal meaning', *Erkenntnis*, 13, 207–24.
Shotter, J. (1981), 'Notes on: Vico, joint action, intentionality, and the making of moral worlds', Paper presented at Colloqium on *Historical Changes in Social Psychology*, Bad Homburg, May 1981.
Spencer-Brown, L. (1969), *Laws of Form*, London: George Allen & Unwin.
Trevarthen, C. and Logotheti, K. (1987), 'First symbols and the nature of human knowledge', Paper presented at the Bergen Workshop on Intersubjectivity and Communication, September 20–26, 1987.
Vološinov, V. N. (1929/1986), *Marxism and the Philosophy of Language*, Cambridge, Mass.: M. I. T. Press.
Vygotsky, L. (1934/1986), *Thought and Language*, Cambridge, Mass.: M. I. T. Press.
Wertsch, J. V. (1979), 'From social interaction to higher psychological processes: A clarification and application of Vygotsky's theory', *Human Development*, 22, 1–22.
Wertsch, J. V. (1988), 'The role of voice in a sociocultural approach to mind', in W. Damon (ed.), *Child Development Today and Tomorrow*, San Francisco: Jossey-Bass.
Winograd, T. (1985), 'Moving the semantic fulcrum', *Linguistics and Philosophy*, 8, 91–104.
Winograd, T. and Flores, C. F. (1986), *Understanding Computers and Cognition: A new foundation for design*. Norwood: Ablex Publications.
Wittgenstein, L. (1962), 'The blue book', in W. Barrett and D. H. Aiken (eds), *Philosophy in the Twentieth Century*, vol. 2, New York: Random House.
Yakubinsky, L. P. (1923/1986), ' O dialogiceskoi reci', in L. P. Yakubinsky, *Izbrannye Raboty*; reprinted in *Yazyk i ego funkcionirovanije*, A. A. Leotiev (ed.), Moscow: Nauka.

5 | Perspectival structure and dynamics in dialogues

Carl F. Graumann

Department of Psychology, University of Heidelberg

Perspectives on the dialogue

The study of language may be approached from different viewpoints. The most familiar broad perspectives are those of *langue* and *parole*. *Parole* – speech, or language use – can itself be approached from different perspectives. One of these, the dialogical, is the perspective adopted in this book. Its prototype, which forms the subject matter of this chapter, is dialogue, the situation of talking together which, in turn, can be considered from different viewpoints. We can focus on the various forms that 'discourse' may take, such as conversation, discussion, debate, dispute or gossip. Or we can turn our attention to the various topics of talk or the social function of different types of dialogue. In this chapter I shall discuss just two perspectives of a dialogue, but first I shall focus briefly on the problem of the conceptualization of two important factors in a dialogue, firstly of *what* is going on in a dialogue. Secondly of *who* is participating in a dialogue.

What is going on in a dialogue

Whatever the different definitions of dialogue may be, there seems to be widespread agreement that the term 'dialogue' refers to the

Part of this chapter is based on a research project, 'Perspectivity and language' made possible by a grant from the *Deutsche Forschungsgemeinschaft* within the context of the Heidelberg/Mannheim *Sonderforschungsbereich* 245 *Sprechen und Sprachverstehen im sozialen Kontext* (*Speech and Language Comprehension in a Social Context*).

togetherness of talking, to the mutuality of exchanging ideas, i.e. to an activity shared by two or more partners. The basic character of this activity is contained in the Greek word, from which our term derives: *dialegesthai*, which is the root of 'dialogos'. This is usually translated as 'conversing' or 'discussing', but it is important to remember its original meaning, which was to speak (and think) together about something in such a way that, while the things about which the speakers are talking are different, yet they become something common *between* them. It is this metaphor of *moving* from two or more positions toward the same place (even if there is agreement to disagree as to what that place should be) that needs further clarification if we want to understand what is meant by 'conversing' or 'exchanging ideas'.

In discourse analysis the question of what is going on in a dialogue is frequently answered by reference to 'utterances'. The term itself implies that inner contents of events, such as ideas or feelings, are expressed by vocal sounds – a useful implication for the psychologist who is interested in the interrelation and interaction between linguistic and mental activities. But in pragmalinguistics the prevailing focus is on utterances as *units* and, consequently, on the rules according to which such units are produced and ordered. Explicitly by analogy with phonemes and morphemes, Pike (1967) introduced the 'uttereme' as a special kind of 'behavioreme'. Although such structuralist notions of units of discourse seem to be out of date, the focus on units and rules is not (Edmonsen, 1981; Taylor and Cameron, 1987). As a basically behavioural unit, 'utterance' refers to a stretch of speech rather than to the act of uttering (see, however, Bakhtin, 1986).

The necessity for discourse analysis is obvious and undisputed (Coulthard, 1977; Henne and Rehbock, 1982). However, there is the danger that by concentrating on the methods of discourse analysis alone, we may neglect the inherent aspects of movement or process that are characteristic of acts of utterance. Those interested in the dynamics of dialogue may be forced to use the tools of discourse analysis, but they must try also to capture the movement involved in talking together.

Interest in the motion occurring in dialogues seems to be lacking altogether in modern models of language processing. Theories of information-processing in language production and comprehension merely account for what is happening between input and output, ignoring what goes on between output and input. Such models are basically monological in kind (Herrmann, 1985; Levelt, 1989).

Who is carrying on a dialogue

The question of who is carrying on a dialogue is easily answered if we look at the literature on discourse analysis. There we are mainly referred to as 'speakers'. Speakers may be categorized according to the following three emphases:

1. The person who *speaks to* the other(s).
2. The person who expects to be and is *spoken to*.
3. The person who is *spoken about* (Jacques, 1979).

Sometimes the person spoken to is categorized as the 'hearer', or 1. and 2. are combined into a 'speaker/hearer'. This is not the place to criticize the reduction of human beings to speakers and hearers – indeed similar reductions are common in the social and behavioural sciences. When the focus of scientific interest is on particular functions we speak of perceivers, of problem-solvers, even of deciders and, most recently, of information-processors. But we should remain conscious of the reductive character of such abstractions, all of which originate in a specific theoretical perspective. The question is, which perspective is the most adequate and productive for a given problem.

If we are interested in the dynamics of dialogue then we may ask ourselves whether speaking (or uttering) and hearing (utterances) constitute an adequate description of the activity of human beings in dialogues. It is not enough if, as is often the case, a speaker/hearer is taken to be a basically independent communication unit (Osgood and Sebeok, 1965), taking turns in 'emitting' or speaking and 'receiving' or hearing messages or utterances. The modern version of this is the information-processing system unit, the most advanced version of which uses an internal partner model, i.e. the partner is interiorized as a subsystem within an integrated speaker–hearer system (Herrmann, 1985). The other person with whom one is in dialogue is aptly named a 'partner', but this term remains theoretically restricted to a cognitive representation in the integrated hearer–speaker system (*ibid.*, pp. 12–14). The original meaning of the word 'partners' as persons sharing something or engaging in a common activity has here been reduced to the representation of two separate units, a consequence of psychological individualism.

A different way of conceptualizing partners in dialogue is in terms of *roles*. This basically dramaturgical notion, favoured by sociologists and (some) social psychologists, presupposes both a context (a social system) and an interrelationship between different roles. Both these features also apply to the dialogue – hence the quite common usage of the phrase 'the role of the speaker (or hearer)' (Graumann and Herrmann, 1989). However, the concept of a role also presupposes a *position* in a social system that can be filled by different individuals. It is difficult to see what the position (in the sociological sense of the word) would represent in the dialogue. Disregarding 'Speaker of the House' and related social positions, it is clear that speakers and hearers are not positions to be filled.

There is a further argument against using the role concept in relation to interlocutors in a dialogue. This derives from the general social-psychological conception that roles carry expectations which others hold about the role occupant's appropriate behaviour, and therefore about the behaviour appropriate to the position presupposed by that role. There are, without doubt, expectations in dialogues that a partner should fulfil according to common postulates or maxims of conversation (Grice, 1975). But this type of appropriateness is conversationally universal rather than position-specific.

Whilst 'partner' seems to be the least restrictive term with which to designate those who engage in a dialogue, it is not specific enough to denote their joint activities and contributions. We need qualifying terms which help us to grasp the characteristic dynamics of dialogues. A very adequate term comes from Bakhtin's literary analyses: *voice* (Bakhtin, 1973; Wertsch, 1987). Voice is consciousness expressed and reaching others, i.e. it is a relational term. A dialogue is a combination of voices, it is polyphonous. The voices in dialogue are persons speaking 'in concert', but a person engaged in a dialogue is not restricted to one voice. He or she may speak with different voices, thus increasing the polyphonous character of dialogues. This differentiation of the dialogue by different but orchestrated voices contributes to its character of *unitas multiplex*. What the metaphor of voice does not allow for, however, is the movement that is implied in the traditional conception of dialogue as an 'exchange of ideas'. The question of what is meant by this figure of speech will be taken up after the concept of perspectivity has been introduced. The discussion of perspectivity presented below is intended to provide further clarification of the structure and dynamics of the dialogue.

The perspectivity of experience

The structure of perspectivity

There is a set of perspectival terms in use in everyday language as well as in several scientific disciplines: perspective, point of view, aspect and horizon are the most common ones. They all refer to different features of a structure of representation which goes back to the Renaissance technique of representing (picturing) objects and scenes so that they appear as if seen from a particular viewpoint or standpoint (Graumann, 1960, 1989). Making use of the later phenomenological explication of perspectivity, we may generalize: from a subject's particular point of view an object is seen in those aspects that correspond to the given viewpoint. But by its very aspectivity the object refers the perceiving subject to further aspects of it, as well as to its immediate surroundings. The house that I view or approach from a given point in space (viewpoint) is present to me in one of its aspects (sides, corners, views) that refers me to the other sides of the house. Wherever I stand, although I see the house *in* one of its aspects, it is never aspects that I see. From whatever position I behold the house I see it in its context – the garden, the street leading to or away from it, the row of houses of which it is one, etc. Since aspects are, by definition, appearances for a subject, the subject is always a constitutive ingredient of perspectival representation without being explicitly 'represented'.

It was principally Husserl (1973) and other phenomenologists and phenomenological psychologists who extended the conception of a perspectival (or horizonal) structure of perceptual experience to all cognitive experience. Also due to them is the idea that an object of thought, such as a problem, is approached from a certain position with respect to which it appears. In other words, it is constituted in one of its aspects, in specific relations to other objects to which the thinking subject is referred within a horizon of comprehension and anticipation.

An example of a person who is presented by various authors in the most disparate aspects or 'faces' is Wilhelm Wundt, one of the founders of modern psychology. He appears as the promoter of a general experimental psychology, which made psychology an individual, independent discipline; or as the most prominent protagonist of a historical and comparative *Völkerpsychologie*, the psychological study of language, mores, myths and law, in which experimentation has no place; or as the philosopher who never wanted psychology to become separated from philosophy; and so on. While it is true that each of these Wundts refers to the identical historical person, each carries its own inner and outer horizon, its own 'thematic field' of relevances (Gurwitsch, 1964).

The dynamics of perspectivity

It is hardly possible to characterize the perspectival structure of experience without referring to its dynamics. Being related intentionally to an object in one of its aspects implies being related referentially to further aspects of that object by a process of mental *locomotion* in a cognitive field. The term locomotion is used here in the sense accorded to it by Lewin (1936), i.e. as any change of position within a field, be it physical, social or conceptual. An aspect is not a sharply bounded part of something. Likewise, the horizon is not a fixed limit, but the line of transition from the perceived to the perceivable, from the known to the knowable, from the actual to the possible, from the given to the new. With each movement of the perceiving or knowing subject the corresponding object changes; the horizon always moves with the subject's locomotion. This incessant locomotion from the actual to the potential is what constitutes the intrinsic dynamics of perspectivity. Potentially, we are always *en route* towards the horizon (van Peursen, 1954); factually, however, we may 'get stuck' within a habitual perspective from which we see 'nothing but' what we are accustomed to seeing (Graumann, 1960). Conditions conducive to cognitive locomotion constitute topics of research into creativity and problem-solving. The creative solution of a problem is very often equivalent to reaching a new perspective.

The reciprocity of perspectives

To take a perspective that is different from the one habitually or presently held is a cognitive skill which is acquired during childhood. According to G. H. Mead (1934), this skill is learned in the context and course of games. When little children play at being parents, teachers or doctors, they are already 'taking roles', i.e. perspectives, as far as they understand them. It is only in rule-governed games that the participating child 'must have the attitude of all the others involved in that game' (*ibid.*, p. 154). Taking the other players' perspectives affects an individual's own acts which, by virtue of this role-taking, are constituted as social acts. To take the attitude of a whole group is a further step towards taking the perspective of 'the generalized other' (*ibid.*).

In the early 1920s the German philosopher and educationalist Theodor Litt (1924), unaware of Mead's (then unpublished) conception of perspective-taking, developed the idea that within each 'perspective of ego' I as an individual am bound to discover 'objects' whose peculiarity it is 'to have a perspective of their own' and which, hence, will have me contained in their perspective (Litt, 1924, p. 33). To know me as contained in another's perspective is to realize that I can and will be seen with different eyes. That is how I can learn to see myself 'differently' (*ibid.*, p. 38). For Litt as much as for Mead, it is the basic *reciprocity of perspectives*, i.e. the mutuality of perspective-taking, that constitutes the conception of the Ego (Litt) or the Self (Mead).

A different conception of reciprocal perspectives is presented by Schutz (1962). His general thesis of the reciprocity of perspectives refers to two pragmatic idealizations: first, that of the 'interchangeability of standpoints'; second, that of the 'congruence of relevance systems'. The former is the assumption that if I were where you are now I would experience things in the same perspective as you do now, and vice versa. The latter is the belief that in spite of all the differences between you and me, due to our different biographies, we can still act together and pursue common goals as if our differences were irrelevant (Schutz and Luckmann, 1973/1974, p. 60). Ultimately, 'the life-world accepted by me as given is also accepted by my fellow-men as given' (*ibid.*, p. 68). (The 'general thesis of the alter ego' was first presented in Schutz, 1932/1967 (p. 106).)

What we learn from the three conceptions of perspectival reciprocity presented by Mead, Litt and Schutz is that perspectives, as inevitable as they may be for human experience, can be transcended, shared or even traded. We learn little from them, however, about how this is accomplished.

Only a few social psychologists have taken up the idea of the reciprocity of perspectives (e.g. Ichheiser, 1943; Laing, Phillipson and Lee, 1966); some have dealt at least with the role of perspective in social judgement (Ostrom, 1966; Ostrom and Upshaw, 1968; Upshaw and Ostrom, 1984; for an overview see Graumann, 1989). But so far the interplay of giving and taking perspective in social interaction has been ignored as a topic of research. In the following section, the focus is on how perspective is presented and accepted, given and taken in linguistic communication.

Perspectivity in dialogues

The triple intentionality of discourse

Uttering something in a dialogue is intentional in three different ways. Borrowing from Karl Bühler (1982) (who in turn goes back to

Plato's conception of language as an *organum*, i.e. as a tool or instrument), we can define speaking as one person's communication with another about something. Phenomenologically, we may recognize in the act of speaking a triple intentionality:

1. In speaking, a person expresses or reveals what he or she is like or has 'in mind', be it ideas, feelings, or intentions.[1]
2. Simultaneously, the speaking person addresses another person, thereby trying to draw the other's attention to what he or she is speaking about.
3. The other person is referred to certain objects or states of affairs by means of speaking.

Going beyond Bühler, whose semiotic organum model is sign-centred, we recognize the triple intentionality of the speech act:

1. The person's (not necessarily conscious) intention to utter his or her thoughts and states of mind.
2. The person's intention to communicate with another person.
3. The person's intention to refer to specific things or events.

It is in this paraphrase of Bühler's model that the perspectivity in dialogue becomes evident. A person referring to an object or state of affairs does so from a particular point of view, in a special sense or relation. When in semantics or in the theory of grammar a distinction is made between the topic of a sentence and its comment (Lyons, 1968, 1977), the topic is that *about which* something is said and the comment *that which* is said about some person or thing. As terms signifying the basic constituents of sentence structure they may suggest that, if we can analytically distinguish between object and viewpoint, the object referred to becomes the topic while the perspective in which a speaker views the object is presented as the comment.

This is indeed often the case. Referring to one individual house I may say, for example:

1. This house is ugly.
2. This house is for sale.
3. This house is the oldest one in the street.

By means of the different comments I am placing my referent in an aesthetic (1.), economic (2.) or historical (3.) perspective. I may also induce such perspectives by means of different topicalizations:

4. The ugliness of this house is an eyesore.
5. The sale of this house has been advertised.
6. The oldest house in the street is here.

It is true that in the comments of 4.–6. some further information is added to the topic, but the perspective in which I want my partner to see the given house may be induced by either topic or comment.

Besides expressing myself and appealing to my partner's attention I refer my partner not only to an object or state of affairs but I also try to make him or her see (understand, conceive, judge, etc.) it the way I do, i.e. from my point of view. 'Reference', therefore, is more than the 'representational' function of signs with respect to non-linguistic entities. It is also, at least in dialogical utterances, the communication of the position from which this entity is seen by a speaker. Only by offering such 'positions-from-which' is the possibility opened for speakers and listeners, for the different voices in a dialogue, jointly to attend a topic from a common 'origo of intersubjectivity' (Rommetveit, 1974, p. 41; 1980).

This joint attention is fully achieved when the triple intentionality of discourse is confirmed by an interlocutor's partner. This triple intentionality is made up of the expression of what a speaker has in mind, the appeal to a listener's attention, and the dual reference to both an object and its mode of apprehension from a given position.[2] That referring in dialogues is a collaborative process has been convincingly demonstrated by Clark and his associates (Clark and Wilkes-Gibbs, 1986; Clark and Schaefer, 1989). The common *origo* is also the point of departure from which interlocutors may jointly move in the cognitive space shared by them (Graumann, 1989) and 'exchange ideas'.

The mutual perspectival evolution of topics in dialogues

We have now reached a point where it should have become evident that perspectivity in language is an intrinsically interactional phenomenon. Whether, beyond the visual sphere, there is something like a purely cognitive, i.e. pre-linguistic, perspective, with its correlative terms of viewpoint and aspects (horizon) of an object, is difficult to decide since almost all we know about our mental structures and processes we have learnt through the medium of language. Whatever I present as my view on a given matter, I offer as a potential perspective for others. Even if the other does not adopt my perspective on a topic, in order to reject it the other speaker must have recognized it as a potential view, i.e. a communicable perspective. Conversely, an interlocutor, in the strict sense of the word, must have the capacity to adopt the perspectives that are proposed by the other participants in a dialogue (Rommetveit, 1974, p. 44). This capacity complements the word knowledge and world knowledge basic to any meaningful language use. Since, however, knowledge always exists in relation to a position (Mannheim, 1936) and 'every constitution of meaning refers back to an individual perspective' (Apel, 1973, p. 98), the capacity to take other persons' perspectives may be considered the elementary communicative competence.

How is this basic mutuality of perspective-taking or rather the give and take of perspectives of a topic manifested in a real dialogue? How can the structure and the dynamics of a dialogue be accounted for in terms of the reciprocity of perspectives? There seems to be more theoretical agreement on this matter than there is empirical evidence.

Resuming our initial questions of what is going on in a dialogue and who is engaging in it, we can now focus on the special issue of what happens to a topic once it has been introduced, i.e. proposed by a speaker and accepted by the other interlocutors. As long as the topic is preserved, i.e. talked about, we may expect something like the 'communicative dynamism' of the Prague School of Linguistics (Daneš, 1974; Eroms, 1986), according to which all utterances are parts of a process of unfolding meaning, but contribute differentially to this evolution.

An empirical illustration

As an example of an unfolding process of accepting, refusing and substituting aspects of a general topic and its subtopics we take the case of a small-group discussion with five French and German interlocutors speaking German. The topic ('Differences in environmental awareness and activities in France and Germany') was introduced and accepted by the group. It was meant to be controversial: for some time, the issue of environmental concern had been discussed differentially and frequently polemically in the French and German media. Many German journalists and politicians had been critical of the French both for their lack of concern for air and water pollution and the seemingly unrestricted growth of their nuclear industry. The French, on the other hand, prided themselves on their expanding clean (nuclear) industry, and ridiculed the mentality of their eastern neighbours who so emphatically bewailed the *Waldster-*

ben (the dying of the forests) in Germany while racing their powerful cars on the *Autobahn* at unlimited speed.

The dialogue that took place was taped and transcribed. The microanalysis of linguistic variables as indicators of perspectives is still in progress.[3] From a first macroanalysis, however, it is possible to portray some of the dynamism due to the unfolding of aspects.[4]

The categories that were used for the structural analysis of the text were as follows:

1. The topic of the dialogue.
2. Aspects of the topic (or subtopics).
4. Explanations of differences.

During the first 20 minutes of what was altogether a 90-minute dialogue on the general topic of the differences in environmental awareness in France and Germany, 3 aspects or facets of this topic were brought up and discussed in terms of 7 explanations for the differences. The thematic sequence of the dialogue is summarized in Table 1 (the explanations are listed separately as being subsequent to the various subtopics).

In order to demonstrate how the general topic is jointly 'processed', either by introducing new perspectives on the topic or by reacting to what had been uttered before, further categories were introduced. These were meant to identify the sequence of arguments in their flow, turns and direction. These categories were as follows:

4. Acceptance (of an argument).
5. Rejection (of an argument).
6. Yes–but reaction (i.e. partial acceptance/rejection).
7. Question (information-seeking utterance).

A summary of one sequence of arguments is given in Table 2. This reveals how some explanations are accepted, i.e. confirmed, some are rejected, e.g. as irrelevant, some are questioned and some are conditionally accepted in typical yes–but responses. But whether accepted, rejected, questioned or qualified, the sequence of arguments reveals that the topic is coherently adhered to. Even a temporary rejection of an argument as 'not relevant' does not break the coherence of the dialogue. As may be gleaned from the transcript, the refusal of one argument is also the challenge to bring in a more 'relevant' one; moreover, the rejected explanation recurs at a later stage of the dialogue.

Whether the group is talking about environmental awareness in

Table 1 The dynamics of a dialogue: perspectival structure in terms of subtopics and explanations of differences

---

1 Topic of the dialogue (between French and German participants): The differences in environmental awareness between France and Germany.

2 Aspects of the topic, as brought up during the dialogue (chronological order):
   (1)* Differences in environmental awareness;
   (6)   Differences in environmental activities;
   (7)   Nuclear plants and the anti-nuclear movement.

3 Explanations offered for differences in environmental awareness (chronological order):
   (2)   Different histories;
   (3)   Differences in population, urban and industrial density and impact;
   (4)   Different attitudes with respect to present and future;
   (5)   Different dispositions to act collectively or individually;
   (8)   Different '1968' traditions: the 'Greens';
   (9)   Centralism in France;
   (10) Different attitudes with respect to capitalism: the ecological movement (cf. 8).

---

*The figures refer to the order of presentation in the full-length transcript.

general, about air and water pollution or about nuclear energy, what they do together is the *dialegesthai*, i.e. the explicating or unfolding of the dialogical 'dis-coursing' and 'dis-cussing' of a shared topic. Sharing, however, does not mean harmony; it may mean tension. Very often the common topic is approached from different, even conflicting viewpoints. Or, an argument may be superficially accepted, but not with the intended meaning.

For a more detailed analysis of the dynamics of dialogue three further pairs of categories were added, to assist in the elucidation of both the position taken by a speaker and the way in which he or she relates to other positions. The categories are thus indicative of (explicit or implicit) attitudinal judgements, and are as follows:

  8. Positive versus negative evaluation (of a position or, generally speaking, the referent of an utterance).
  9. Identifying with versus distancing from (a position or attitude).
10. Emphasizing versus de-emphasizing (a position or attitude).

The following examples taken from the transcript illustrate the usefulness of our categories for the reconstruction of the perspectival dynamics of a dialogue, i.e. the setting, taking or refusing to take the interlocutor's perspective on the shared topic.

A French discussant tries to account for the differences in ecological awareness in the two countries by reference to their respective histories. Her argument is that the discontinuity of German history in 1945 was a chance to reconsider old ideas critically and to develop new ones. A German partner, while agreeing that the Germans do have the problem of coping with their recent (Nazi) history, dismisses the historical argument as irrelevant for the topic under discussion. But a few minutes later, when the role of the political parties is discussed, it is the same German interlocutor who wonders why, in France, 1968 has not resulted in an ecological movement, as it has in Germany.

The act of making an aspect a subject of discourse is an act of selection and an effort to structure (control) the next phase of the dialogue in accordance with one's *values*. The perspective in which a speaker presents a topic and which the hearer is invited to take is rarely evaluatively neutral. In most cases, the aspects that we select are positive or negative evaluations of the object of reference. In any event, they will be evaluated by our partners.

For Nietzsche, the most profound philosopher of the perspectivity of life, perspectives are intrinsically evaluative. To posit values is to set perspectives and horizons (Nietzsche, 1980, p. 20; Graumann, 1960, pp. 38–44). In a dialogue, the perspective I present is for me (and for the time being) a preferred perspective. Yours will be too, from your point of view. What we call the *divergence of perspectives* (Graumann, 1989; Mummendey, Linneweber and Löschper, 1984; Mummendey and Otten, 1989) is basically a difference of valuation. That is why utterances reveal a speaker's perspective not only by the more or less explicit reference to a standpoint, but also by direct or indirect evaluations.

Discussing, for example, the *Waldsterben*, a French interlocutor may explicitly state that from her point of view it is incomprehensible that the Germans, who keep lamenting the dying of their forests, are unwilling to introduce a speed limit on their *Autobahnen*. But within the context of air pollution and acid rain, the mere reference to unlimited speed is in itself a critical utterance. The same applies in the taped dialogue to a German speaker's reference to the French lack of concern over their increasing production of nuclear energy, when the topic under discussion is environmental awareness. The conclusion of his practical syllogism, namely that the French ought to be concerned, cannot be endorsed by his French partners since they do not share his premiss that 'everybody knows about the sickness and the grass getting brown.'

Table 2 The dynamics of a dialogue: the perspectival development of the topic

	Germans		French
(1)	*E*(nvironmental) *awareness*, still weak in G, in F even weaker.	acc →	People in F are not concerned by the Rhine, Loire, Chernobyl catastrophes.
(2)			The difference may have to do with Germany's *past*:
	This is a different topic.	rej ←	The reconstruction after World War II.
(3)			More urban and industrial *density* in G. Everything is so narrow. People need woods and fresh air. In F there is more wilderness. You can get there by bike. In G you need the car.
	But there are high-density areas in F. There should be *more concern* in F. More actions.	y/b ←	In F it is not so necessary to protect nature
(2)		y/b →	Yes, but the *past* is also important. F has an old tradition. Things change gradually.
	I doubt it. Look how little the G have learnt from their past. Take rearmament.	rej ←	There was no break with our past. In G there was something new.
(3)	But, irrespective of history, there is the *immediate impact*, such as the salination of the Rhine (by the F). But the F are not worried. Why?		
(4)	Perhaps it has to do with a different *attitude towards the future*; the F tend to enjoy the present and do not care about the future. Is this not a stereotype?	acc → ? ←	There may be a great difference. We F enjoy life, in G life is more 'intellectualized'.
(5)			The F do not fight so much *collectively*, in demonstrations like the G who take to the streets. The F act more *individually*.

Table 2 The dynamics of a dialogue: the perspectival development of the topic *cont.*

	Germans			French
		rej		*In F, we do not do much;*
(6)	I must contradict: in G far too little is being done.	←		*in G, they do too much.* Not enough Greens in F, but in G there are many. In G people sort out three different kinds of garbage. In F we would find this too arduous.
(7)	In F you have so many *nuclear plants*. The F do not do anything about them in spite of the great danger. Everybody knows about the amount of sickness and the grass getting brown. This ought to concern the F.	? →		Never heard about such things in the newspapers.
(8)	This is not a matter of information. In F no ecological movement developed from the *'68 movement*; why? In G most 'sixty-eighters' ended up in the ecological movement. The difference is incomprehensible.	rej ←		
(9)	Perhaps F has been centralized for too long. Centralism fosters passivity.	acc →		Possibly, people expect more from Paris than from themselves.
(10)	In G, an attitude *opposed to capitalism* with its tendency to ignore the environment. Perhaps in F people do not feel restricted.	acc →		People in F feel far away from the State and from Paris. Every man for himself!

Legend

G	German(s), Germany	→	responses	y/b	yes-but response
F	French, France	acc	acceptance	?	questioning
E	environment(al)	rej	rejection	(1)	figures refer to the order of presentation (first mention)

Sometimes the means of perspectival evaluation are too subtle for discovery by macroanalysis. Thus, distancing from and identifying with a position are dynamically essential modes of structuring a cognitive space with respect to different positions. A German speaker, for instance, may be 'totally unable to understand' that the French do not get excited over the pollution of the rivers Rhine and Loire. He explicitly distances himself from the 'incomprehensible' French indifference. On the other hand, a French interlocutor, under the impression that in Germany the density of buildings is very high, expresses her understanding for the Germans' dependence on cars: they need to get out to the woods for fresh air. But why at unlimited speed?

Sometimes the distancing or identifying attitude is recognizable in the (perhaps involuntary) choice of pronouns or of personal versus impersonal forms of immediacy versus non-immediacy (Wiener and Mehrabian, 1968; Graumann and Wintermantel, 1989). As Marisa Zavalloni (1971) has demonstrated, there are two grammatically distinct ways of referring to one's own group: one uses the identificatory 'we', the other the distancing 'they' or 'people'. In the taped dialogue we discover this differential reference to one's own group by means of which a distancing or identifying attitude is revealed. In terms of perspective theory an interlocutor either takes the perspective of others or merely indicates the difference between his or her own and the others' views.

This differential usage in speakers' references to their own group is evident in our Franco-German dialogue. For example, a German speaker criticizes the Germans who, after Chernobyl, 'were so stupid that they went to Alsace in order to buy non-contaminated cabbage . . .'. Here, evidently, the speaker distances himself from 'the Germans', just as a French speaker does in the following sentence about the French, referring to them as 'people': '*People* don't care about the environment, maybe *people* care about their own gardens . . .'. Conversely, the same French speaker identifies with the French when discussing garbage disposal. She states: 'People (in Germany) very often keep three (separate) kinds of garbage in their kitchen . . . . *We* don't do it that way and maybe *we* couldn't do it in France. *We* would find it too arduous.'

Conclusion

All through the recorded dialogue the theme of the difference in ecological awareness between the French and the Germans is adhered to by the interlocutors. It is true that this dialogue is a debate rather than a conversation. Its controversial character is evident on every page of the transcript, not only between the French and the German partners but also within the two national groups. There is, however, from the beginning to the end of the dialogue, agreement on the difference (in ecological awareness) which constitutes and preserves the *identity* of the topic. This identity is the common ground on which the dialogue partners move. It is the *sine qua non* of the locomotion of the *dialegesthai*. According to the theory of perspectivity, different dialogue partners approach a common topic from different positions, which amounts to the fact that they (perceive and) thematize different aspects of their common topic.

What makes up the dynamics of a dialogue is the effort of the different interlocutors to bring their own perspective to bear, i.e. to succeed in setting a given perspective for partners to take up, at least for the next few turns. In our sample dialogue it happens several times that an interlocutor succeeds in setting his or her perspective on the common topic without or against the resistance of others. Resistance may be the flat rejection of a view as irrelevant. More often, however, the dynamics of the dialogue are fed by subtle qualifications of the perspective presented: it is accepted, but evaluated differently by moving to a related aspect within the horizon of comprehension.

When, for instance, the theme of the nuclear industry is struck up by a German interlocutor it is from a critical viewpoint: why is there no strong anti-nuclear movement in France as there is in Germany? From a different point of view, by contrast, nuclear energy is seen as 'clean', as it does not cause the air pollution brought about by the use of fossil energy. Moreover, a French interlocutor reminds her German partners that the Germans buy cheap French electricity, i.e. from nuclear plants. This ultimately means that the French interlocutor has accepted the nuclear issue as a facet of the topic 'ecological awareness', but has set this subtopic in a different (and differently valued) perspective. A similar shift of perspective happens when the above-mentioned German complaint about the *Waldsterben* is commented upon by a French partner in terms of air pollution as co-determined by the German habit of driving at unlimited speed.

What in linguistics, since Grice (1975), has been termed conversational implicatures refers partly to such inferences as may be drawn from the horizon of meaning in which each topic is perspectivally perceived or, rather, understood. These implicatures contribute to the dynamics of a dialogue. Implications of what has been uttered are not only discovered by a speaker's hearer. Often enough it is the speaker him- or herself who, while speaking, or rather while listening to his or her own speaking, detects implicit meanings in his or her utterance that were not meant to be expressed but, once recognized, may be taken into account. An example of this is the German dialogue partner who, while criticizing the French for their lack of environmental concern, realizes that in Germany too ecological awareness is far from satisfactory. Or the French interlocutor who, while acknowledging that the French do not do enough in terms of environmental activities, realizes that they have at least started to do something to protect their environment. Clearly there was a good chance by now of the differences between the two sides being resolved. Generally speaking, as the perspectival unfolding of a topic proceeds, between and within the partners of a dialogue, the implications of a given aspect are progressively explicated.

The above examples serve to illustrate the point that the dynamics of a dialogue are to be found not only in the different perspectives that stem from the fact that different interlocutors interact, but also from the possibility that one and the same speaker may contribute different voices to the dialogue: positive and negative ones, pros and cons, emphatic or reserved, voices to keep one's distance from and voices to identify with somebody or something. The polyphony of a dialogue originates in the variety of voices both between and within interlocutors. It is with reference to this polyphony of voices that we should answer the question of *who* is carrying on a dialogue.

Speaking in a different voice is not restricted to rare instances of conversion. It is the ordinary case with *dialegein*: when in conversation I will anticipate differing viewpoints or objections from the person I am talking to and will try to incorporate them into my own speech. Sometimes I will explicitly contrast differing viewpoints: 'on the one hand . . . on the other hand', 'in one respect . . .', 'for one thing . . . for another thing', 'from my point of view . . . from yours', etc. Or I will raise self-objections, self-criticisms, introduce hedges and reservations. Often my mental reservations become manifest only in qualifying conjunctions and adverbs like but, though, yet and however.

The whole repertoire of rhetorics is available for the expression of the multiperspectivity of cognition. Michael Billig (1987, p. 49) summarizes this: it has always been the rhetorical approach that 'stresses the two-sidedness of human thinking and of our conceptual capacities', i.e. the dialogical character of human cognition. This is why the proper place to study cognition is in the dialogue rather than in monological information-processing. I concur with Markus and Zajonc (1985, pp. 212f.) who, discussing the communicative aspect of social cognition, criticize 'a unilateral input/output paradigm that stops short of reciprocity', and who dare to predict that:

> It is likely that in the near future the major new method of studying social cognition and cognition in general will be the dialogue . . . individual subjects in interaction . . . may disclose a great deal of context and structure of their own cognitions and help reveal the cognitions of others. (*ibid.*)

For social psychologists, who do not shy away from the study of interaction, a decision to study cognition in dialogues implies the readiness, at last, to include the everyday use of language in their field of study and, with the help of language psychologists, to develop and refine methods that are capable of capturing the reciprocity and multiperspectivity of dialogical interaction.

Notes

1. For Bühler (1982) the expressive function of signs does not refer to everything a 'sender' may have 'in mind', but rather reveals inner states like feelings, moods or the whole of character or personality. Bühler's favourite correlate of expression is *Innerlichkeit*, the spiritual world within a person.
2. It would be possible to categorize the communication of a person's perspective as the 'expression' of what the person has in mind, i.e. with respect to an object or state of affairs. But this would be a significant redefinition of the term as established by Bühler (see note 1).
3. Dependent linguistic variables indicative of the perspective taken by a speaker have been developed and validated in a series of experiments on perspective structure in language production and comprehension (Graumann and Sommer, 1989).
4. For the transcription and evaluation of the French–German dialogue I owe all of the data and some of the categories to the co-operative help of C. M. Sommer, E. Bröstler, B. Freitag, H. Jokisch, R. Höer, G. Klemp and M. Kraus. A full report on this study will be published elsewhere.

References

Apel, K. O. (1973), *Transformation der Philosophie*, vol. II: *Das Apriori der Kommunikationsgemeinschaft*, Frankfurt: Suhrkamp.
Bakhtin, M. (1973), *Problems of Dostoevsky's Poetics*, Ann Arbor: Ardis.
Bakhtin, M. (1986), *Speech Genres and Other Late Essays*, C. Emerson and M. Holquist (eds), Austin: University of Texas Press.

Billig, M. (1987), *Arguing and Thinking: A rhetorical approach to social psychology*, Cambridge: Cambridge University Press.
Bühler, K. (1982), 'The axiomatization of the language sciences', in R. E. Innis (ed.), *Karl Bühler. Semiotic Foundations of Language Theory*, New York and London: Plenum.
Clark, H. H. and Wilkes-Gibbs, D. (1986), 'Referring as a collaborative process', *Cognition*, 22, 1–39.
Clark, H. H. and Schaefer, E. F. (1989), 'Collaborating on contributions to conversations', in R. Dietrich and C. F. Graumann (eds), *Language Processing in Social Context*, Amsterdam: North Holland.
Coulthard, M. (1977), *An Introduction to Discourse Analysis*, London: Longman.
Daneš, F. (ed.) (1974), *Papers on Functional Sentence Perspective*, Prague: Prague Academia.
Edmonsen, C. (1981), *Spoken Discourse*, London: Longman.
Eroms, H. W. (1986), *Funktionale Satzperspektive*, Tübingen: Niemeyer.
Graumann, C. F. (1960), *Grundlagen einer Phänomenologie und Psychologie der Perspektivität*, Berlin: de Gruyter.
Graumann, C. F. (1989), 'Perspective setting and taking in verbal interaction', in R. Dietrich and C. F. Graumann (eds), *Language Processing in Social Context*, Amsterdam: North Holland.
Graumann, C. F. and Herrmann, T. (eds) (1989), *Speakers: The role of the listener*, Clevedon: Multilingual Matters.
Graumann, C. F. and Sommer, C. M. (1989), 'Perspective structure in language production and comprehension', in C. F. Graumann and T. Herrmann (eds), *Speakers: The role of the listener*, Clevedon: Multilingual Matters.
Graumann, C. F. and Wintermantel, M. (1989), 'Discriminatory speech-acts: A functional approach', in D. Bar-Tal, C. F. Graumann, A. W. Kruglanski and W. Stroebe (eds), *Stereotyping and Prejudice: Changing conceptions*, New York: Springer-Verlag.
Grice, H. P. (1975), 'Logic and conversation', in P. Cole and J. L. Morgan (eds), *Syntax and Semantics*, vol. 3: *Speech Acts*, New York: Academic Press.
Gurwitsch, A. (1964), *The Field of Consciousness*, Pittsburgh: Duquesne University Press.
Henne, H. and Rehbock, H. (1982), *Einführung in die Gesprächsanalyse*, 2nd edition, Berlin: de Gruyter.
Herrmann, T. (1985), *Allgemeine Sprachpsychologie*, München: Urban & Schwarzenberg.
Husserl, E. (1973), *Experience and Judgment*, Evanston, Ill.: Northwestern University Press.
Ichheiser, G. (1943), 'Structure and dynamics of interpersonal relations', *American Sociological Review*, 8, 302–05.
Jacques, F. (1979), *Dialogiques*, Paris: Presses Universitaires de France.
Laing, R. D., Phillipson, H. and Lee, A. R. (1966), *Interpersonal Perception*, London: Tavistock.
Levelt, W. J. M. (1989), *Speaking: From intention to articulation*, Cambridge, Mass.: MIT Press.
Lewin, K. (1936), *Principles of Topological Psychology*, New York: McGraw-Hill.
Litt, T. (1924), *Individuum und Gemeinschaft*, 2nd edition, Leipzig: B. G. Teubner.

Lyons, J. (1968), *Introduction to Theoretical Linguistics*, Cambridge: Cambridge University Press.
Lyons, J. (1977), *Semantics*, 2 vols, Cambridge: Cambridge University Press.
Mannheim, K. (1936), *Ideology and Utopia: An introduction to the sociology of knowledge*, trans. L. Wirth and E. Shils, New York: Harcourt Brace.
Markus, H. and Zajonc, R. B. (1985), 'The cognitive perspective in social psychology', in G. Lindzey and E. Aronson (eds), *Handbook of Social Psychology* (3rd edition), vol. I, New York: Random House.
Mead, G. H. (1934), *Mind, Self, and Society*, Chicago: University of Chicago Press.
Mummendey, A., Linneweber, V. and Löschper, G. (1984), 'Aggression: From act to interaction', in A. Mummendey (ed.), *Social Psychology of Aggression*, Berlin: Springer-Verlag.
Mummendey, A. and Otten, S. (1989), 'Perspective-specific differences in the segmentation and evaluation of aggressive interaction sequences', *European Journal of Social Psychology*, 19, 23–40.
Nietzsche, F. (1980), 'Menschliches, Allzumenschliches', *Sämtliche Werke. Kritische Studienausgabe in 15 Bänden*, V. G. Colli and M. Montinari (eds), vol. 2, München: Deutscher Taschenbuch Verlag.
Osgood, C. E. and Sebeok, T. A. (eds) (1965), *Psycholinguistics: A survey of theory and research problems*, Bloomington: Indiana University Press.
Ostrom, T. M. (1966), 'Perspective as an intervening construct in the judgement of attitude statements', *Journal of Personality and Social Psychology*, 3, 135–44.
Ostrom, T. M. and Upshaw, H. S. (1968), 'Psychological perspective and attitude change', in A. G. Greenwald, T. C. Brock and T. M. Ostrom (eds), *Psychological Foundations of Attitudes*, New York: Academic Press.
Peursen, C. A. van (1954), 'L'horizon', *Situation*, 1, 204–34.
Pike, K. (1967), *Language in Relation to a Unified Theory of Human Behavior* (2nd edition), The Hague: Mouton.
Rommetveit, R. (1974), *On Message Structure: A framework for the study of language and communication*, London: Wiley.
Rommetveit, R. (1980), 'On "meanings" of acts and what is meant and made known by what is said in a pluralistic social world', in M. Brenner (ed.), *The Structure of Action*, Oxford: Blackwell.
Schutz, A. (1932/1967), *Der sinnhafte Aufbau der sozialen Welt*, Wien: Springer; reprinted 1960. Trans. by G. Walsh and F. Lehnert as *The Phenomenology of the Social World*, 1967 Evanston, Ill.: Northwestern University Press; London: Heinemann Educational Books, 1972.
Schutz, A. (1962), *Collected Papers*, vol. 1, The Hague: Nijhoff.
Schutz, A. and Luckmann, T. (1973/1974), *The Structures of the Life-World*, trans. R. M. Zaner and H. T. Engelhardt jr, 1973 Evanston, Ill.: Northwestern University Press; London: Heinemann, 1974.
Taylor, T. J. and Cameron, D. (1987), *Analysing Conversation – Rules and Units in the Structure of Talk*, Oxford: Pergamon.
Upshaw, H. S. and Ostrom, T. M. (1984), 'Psychological perspective in attitude research', in J. R. Eiser (ed.), *Attitudinal Judgment*, New York: Springer-Verlag.
Wertsch, J. (1987), 'The role of voice in a socio-cultural approach to mind', in W. Damon (ed.), *Child Development Today and Tomorrow*, San Francisco: Jossey-Bass.

Wiener, M. and Mehrabian, A. (1968), *Language Within Language: Immediacy, a channel in verbal communication*, New York: Appleton-Century-Crofts.

Zavalloni, M. (1971), 'Cognitive processes and social identity through focussed introspection', *European Journal of Experimental Social Psychology*, 1 (2), 235–60.

PART II
Specific aspects of dialogical dynamics

6 | A three-step process as a unit of analysis in dialogue

Ivana Markovà
Department of Psychology, University of Stirling

Introduction

Students of dialogue will, sooner or later in their research, come to face the following question: in what ways can one subdivide a dialogue in order to identify meaningful units for its analysis? In other words, what can be taken as an appropriate analytical starting point: a sentence, a turn, an utterance, a question–answer, or a unit based on more turns? Even if this question is not stated by the researcher explicitly, it is still likely to be present implicitly and will, therefore, have to be addressed. Let us consider some possible answers.

Using a *single utterance* or a *turn* (these are not equivalent) as the unit of analysis, the researcher might conceive of a dialogue as consisting of utterance sequences or of turn sequences, with a single utterance or single turn being a meaningful unit in its own right. For example, the researcher's problem could be that of identifying the dominant topics in a dialogue. For this purpose, he or she would classify single utterances into categories according to their contents. Another kind of presupposition based on a single utterance as the unit of analysis has been made by speech act theory. Speech act theory is based on the hypothesis that speaking a language consists of performing intentional rule-governed acts such as making statements or promises, giving commands and so on (Searle, 1969). This

---

I would like to thank Klaus Foppa, Per Linell, Ragnar Rommetveit and Colin Wright for their comments on previous versions of this chapter.

hypothesis further states that whatever can be meant can be said and that the minimal units of linguistic communication are single speech acts (see also Labov and Fanshel, 1977; Kreckel, 1981).

Socially oriented researchers emphasize the interactive nature of dialogue. For them, the use of isolated utterances or single speech acts as the units of analysis is neither theoretically nor methodologically acceptable because it fails to acknowledge the embeddedness of single utterances in social interaction and social situations (Schegloff and Sacks, 1973; Levinson, 1981; Atkinson and Heritage, 1984). Assuming such embeddedness of utterances, social psychologists use *the interlocutors' interactive turns* as the units of analysis. Turn-taking is considered to play an essential role in structuring people's social interactions in terms of control and regulation of conversation, and its mechanism has been carefully explored (e.g. Wiemann, 1985). In a similar vein, conversation analysts attempt to understand sequences of utterances as the products of interaction (Atkinson and Heritage, 1984). The units of analysis in conversation are defined as suitable adjacency pairs such as question–answer or statement–comment (Schegloff and Sacks, 1973; Schegloff, 1984). For example, Pomerantz (1984) explores speakers' strategies of soliciting responses to their question or assertion if their interlocutors fail to provide any.

A unit of analysis consisting of the triad *initiative, response* and *feedback* has been used by Sinclair and Coulthard (1975) in their classroom studies of interactions. These authors have argued that the addition of a third step, i.e. that of feedback, to mutual turn-taking, is an important educational device: the teacher should provide pupils with feedback evaluating their performance. Conversation analysts such as Schegloff and Sacks (1973), Schegloff (1979), Jefferson (1989) and Drew (1990) also argue for a tripartite analysis to be used, at least in some cases. For example, after the second speaker's turn, the first speaker may correct or repair any misunderstanding in the second speaker's turn by displaying a 'third position repair' (Schegloff, 1979). Moreover, Jefferson (1989) observes that many lists of items in natural conversation occur in three parts. She gives numerous examples showing that the third in a list of items serves the purpose of a general 'completer'. For instance, one interlocutor says something that is commented on or disputed by the other interlocutor and, as a result, the first interlocutor completes or summarizes the preceding communicative exchange. The third item thus appears to serve as a means of managing a discord by reformulating what the two opposing parties have already stated, and by so doing it enables a smooth transition to take place from one speaker to the next. According to this view, tripartition facilitates the 'poetics' of natural talk and it occurs most often in puns, jokes, estimates and exaggerations. In general, some conversation analysts maintain that tripartition is a structural principle according to which conversational sequencing is organized and interactional negotiations take place (Jefferson, 1989).

All the approaches we have discussed so far are based on attempts *physically* to subdivide a dialogue in a meaningful manner into small units that have actual boundaries separating one unit from the other. For example, in the case of single turns as units of analysis, the boundaries between turns are defined by the switch from the one interlocutor to the other. Adjacency pairs as units of analysis are defined as two physical turns, e.g. question and answer, greeting and greeting, or topic and comment. In the case of tripartite units one looks for three turns, the third being a feedback from the previous two.

The primary concern of analysis based on physical subdivision of a dialogue or its parts into dialogical units is to answer certain questions about the organization, patterns and rules guiding the sequencing of a dialogue. While this kind of analysis has enhanced knowledge in these subjects, it is not really suitable for dealing with other subjects, for example with problems concerning the embeddedness of utterances in their linguistic and social contexts, the speakers' perspectives and other issues of the dynamics of dialogue, because it is not primarily concerned with dialogical interdependencies.

In order to capture the dynamic characteristics of dialogue I shall take a different approach. Adopting the epistemological position of *dialogism* (see Markovà, this volume, Introduction), I shall argue for units of analysis that are *primarily conceptual and epistemological* in character. Only when the units of analysis are defined conceptually, can one, secondarily, search for their physical expression in speech, and in dialogue in particular. The units of analysis for which I shall argue are conceptually based on *three-step processes*, and they are derived from co-genetic logic (see Markovà, this volume, Introduction, p. 14; Rommetveit, this volume, Chapter 4). The basic assumption of this approach is that every message is embedded in its linguistic and social contexts and that it is both past- and future-oriented, i.e. it is both retroactive and proactive. My arguments for three-step processes will be divided into two sections. In the first section I shall discuss the ideas of mutuality and internal relations between speech expressions in given concrete situations and their embeddedness in language as such. This idea is fundamental for the analysis of speech based on three-step processes which is discussed in the second part of this chapter.

The logic of internal relations

Internal relations are an inherent part of the subject matter of a logic that has been called *dialectic*, or *dialogical* or *co-genetic*. Dialectic logic can be traced back to the philosophers of the eighteenth and early nineteenth centuries. Among these, Fichte (1794/1970) and Hegel (1812–16) postulated the basic principle of dialectic logic as being a triadic development of phenomena *related internally* as parts of a whole. According to this logic of triadic development, every phenomenon, be it an organism, a speech action or a single word, has its 'outside'. The phenomenon and its 'outside' complement each other, both being parts of the same whole. They are defined in terms of each other, just like figure and ground, and each determines what the other is and how it functions in time (Harris, 1983, p. 30). These characteristics distinguish *internally related* phenomena from those *related externally*. External relations are modelled by the mathematical or formal logic of truth-values. According to this logic, elementary propositions, for example 'it is windy', 'it is rainy', can be combined by means of logical connectives, e.g. 'and', into more complex propositions, e.g. 'it is windy and rainy'. The connective 'and' thus represents an external relation between the two elementary propositions without modifying them in any way. In general, external relations do not affect the content of propositions and leave their truth-value unchanged. In contrast, a phenomenon and its 'outside' that are internally related cannot be separated from each other in the way that externally related elements can. If internally related phenomena are separated from each other, they cease to be what they were. It is internal relations of this kind, binding together the element and its opposite (its 'outside'), that give rise to the well-known triad of *thesis, antithesis* and *synthesis* (Fichte, 1794/1970). Recently, and as Rommetveit maintains, a similar kind of logic, a so-called *co-genetic logic*, has been established by Spencer-Brown (1969) and Herbst (1987a, 1987b), although seemingly without the influence of Fichte and Hegel (see the discussion of this question by Rommetveit, this volume, Chapter 4).

The logic of internal relations underlies the co-development of all mutually interdependent phenomena, for example, of the individual and its environment. The two, individual and environment, come into existence together. What had existed before the individual in question emerged, was only the potential environment of a potential individual (Gibson, 1979; Marková, 1987), but not the actual environment of anything. 'Individual' and 'environment', properly understood, are relational terms, and one component in the dyad formed of the two cannot be properly understood in isolation from the other. The intelligibility of the term 'individual' in the dyad 'individual–environment' is dependent on the intelligibility of its counterpart, 'environment'. If one component of the dyad undergoes change or development, the logic of their relationship is such that the other component also undergoes change or development: the two components of a dyad develop in unison. For example, in this process individuals respond to or are sensitive to particular aspects of their environment. They do not just adapt themselves to their 'outside' but mould it to suit themselves through their particular activities: birds build nests and people construct aeroplanes, each species using appropriate materials from their environments. The environment so changed through such activities in turn alters the moulders themselves.

The idea of internal relations between phenomena therefore implies three-step processes: as the two phenomena interact, co-determining each other, they give rise to a new, i.e. a third, phenomenon that is qualitatively different from the two constitutive ones.

Among the first scholars who contributed to the formulation of the idea of three-step processes in language was Wilhelm von Humboldt. He pointed to the internal relations that exist between language as a social possession and language as an individual creation. As a social possession language may be conceived as a stock of words and a system of rules which, over the course of millennia, has become so stable as to exert an invisible power over individual human beings. At the same time, however, each person expresses him- or herself in language as if it peculiarly belongs to him or her. In this sense language lives only through actual speech and individual comprehension. Consequently, although the power of language on the individual is far greater than that of the individual on language, each individual, nevertheless, does potentially effect language change. This is so, Humboldt argued, because it is only in the individual that language acquires its finite characteristics:

> Nobody conceives in a given word exactly what his neighbour does, and the ever so slight variation skitters through the entire language like concentric ripples over the water. All understanding is simultaneously a noncomprehension, all agreement in ideas and emotions is at the same time a divergence. In the manner in which language is modified by each individual there is revealed, in contrast to its previously expounded potency, a power of man over it. (Humboldt, 1836/1971, p. 43)

For example, in naming a horse 'a horse' everyone means the same kind of animal, but each person has his or her idiosyncratic concept of a horse that overlaps, rather than is identical to, those of other persons (Humboldt, 1836/1971, I, p. ccviii). In terms of a three-step process, every speech action is the result of interaction between the individual's idiosyncratic language expression and language as a collective possession. Thus, Humboldt argued that language is both a permanent and a transient phenomenon: permanent in the sense that it is a constant possession of people, and transient because it continuously changes and develops. In other words, just as every living organism contributes to the life of its species, so each speech action contributes to the language that is in the possession of the community of which he or she is a member.

Following Humboldt, one of the Prague School semioticians, Sergej Karcevskij (1929/1982),[1] argued that language operates between two poles that can be characterized as collective–individual, abstract–concrete or stable–dynamic. One pole cannot be reduced to the other, but they are dialectically related through their similarity to and difference from the other. This polarity is best expressed in Karcevskij's theory of asymmetric dualism, according to which each linguistic sign is, simultaneously, potentially both a *homonym*, i.e. can apply to a variety of situations, and a *synonym*, i.e. can imply the use of other signs that could be meaningfully applied in the given situation. The actual use of the linguistic sign results in what Karcevskij called a *tertium comparationis*, i.e. the sign relates both to the common use of the term and to the new situation in which it is used; a *tertium comparationis* 'motivates the new value of the old sign' (*ibid.*, p. 52). If we adopt Karcevskij's position, *tertium comparationis* can be viewed as the third step in a three-step process in which a new linguistic sign is produced when a potential or conventional sign is applied in a concrete situation. According to this view homonymic and synonymic series remain infinitely open: there are always new possible situations in which a given linguistic sign can be used and at the same time there are always new possible associations of one linguistic sign with others.

Such ideas were taken for granted by the Prague semioticians who, in contrast to Saussure (1916/1960), argued that pure a-developmental synchronic structure is an illusion. Instead, 'every synchronic system has its past and its future as inseparable structural elements of the system . . . every system necessarily exists as an evolution

1. I am grateful to Jim Wertsch for bringing to my attention the English publication (1982) of Karcevskij's (1929) paper on asymmetric dualism.

whereas, on the other hand, evolution is inescapably of a systematic nature' (Tynjanov and Jakobson, 1928/1972, p. 82). An utterance separated from its context in a dialogue no longer has the meaning it had as a part of that dialogue. On its own the utterance only has a meaning potentiality and its proper meaning can be determined only in relation to the particular context to which it belongs (see also Vološinov, 1973; Rommetveit, 1974).

While semioticians like Mukařovský, Karcevskij and Jakobson were developing their ideas in Prague, Bakhtin (1981), in Soviet Russia, was arguing in a similar manner. Words, he pointed out, do not live in some neutral and impersonal language but in other people's mouths and contexts, and as expressions of their intentions. Words are 'appropriated' by the individuals who use them (see also Wertsch, this volume, Chapter 3). A word becomes 'one's own' only when one populates it with one's own intention, own accent, adapting it to one's own semantic and expressive intention. Moreover, the meanings of words are co-determined by interlocutors. Bakhtin (Vološinov, 1973) persistently referred to a word as a two-sided act, as a bridge cast between speaker and listener.

The idea that carrying on a conversation necessarily involves an internal relation between individual perspective and common perspective was also argued by George Herbert Mead (1927/1982). Such an internal relation between individual and common perspective develops as the individual learns to take the attitude of others towards him- or herself, i.e. learns to view him- or herself as an object through the eyes of others. As Mead argues, it is only when the individual is able to take on the attitude of the other person and, more broadly, the attitude of the generalized other, that he or she is able to respond to him- or herself through the attitude of the group or the community. Just as individual and common perspective are jointly determined, so the meanings of words and gestures in a conversation are the results of a collaborative process on the part of the involved individuals.

One can see from this brief historical account that the dialogical conception of language, i.e. dialogical in the epistemological sense, has been adopted by scholars from different traditions and backgrounds. It is implicit in the conceptions of these scholars that the actual use of language in concrete situations is the result of some kind of three-step process. They have all viewed speech as dynamic in terms of temporal and internal relations between language as a social possession and the individual's activity, and the meanings of words and utterances as mutually co-determined by the interlocutors.

Different levels of three-step processes

Our discussion of internal relations and three-step processes in the previous section has included two kinds of speech embeddedness. The first has concerned the embeddedness of speech in concrete situations. This means that *what is said* is viewed as a result of the interaction between two socio-linguistic poles: that of language as a *meaning potential*, i.e. as a public possession providing the possibility of having a *concrete meaning*; and that of speech as an idiosyncratic expression of the individual who implements it in the here-and-now. The second kind of embeddedness concerns the view that *what is said* is part of a continuous process in verbal communication in which the speaker and the listener jointly construct the meaning of a linguistic item:

> Each and every word expresses the 'one' in relation to the 'other'. I give myself verbal shape from another's point of view of the community to which I belong. A word is a bridge thrown between myself and another. If one end of the bridge depends on me, then the other depends on my addressee. A word is territory shared by both addresser and addressee, by the speaker and his inter-locutor.
> (Vološinov, 1973, p. 86)

It is in this sense that one can say about a word or utterance that it is both retroactive and proactive, self- and other-oriented, decoding and encoding. It is these pairs of dyadic features that make the word or utterance 'a bridge thrown between myself and another' and thus a connecting bond embedded in a dialogical process.

In dialogue as face-to-face immediate interaction both kinds of embeddedness co-exist and either of them can become the basis for a three-step unit of analysis. In the following section we shall consider some examples of such units.

A three-step unit as a turn

In Linell's analysis of *interactional dominance* (Linell, Gustavsson and Juvonen, 1988; Linell, this volume, Chapter 7), each turn, conceptually, is viewed as a result of some degree of initiative and response. By looking at initiative and response in each turn in terms of maintenance and changing of topic by the interlocutors, the researcher's problem is to identify the features of interactional dominance. Each turn has the characteristics of a three-step process, each turn being the result of interaction between some initiative and some response. As Linell (this volume, Chapter 7) claims, each turn or utterance is Janus-like, i.e. it is potentially directed simultaneously towards the past and towards the future. The retroactive feature of the turn or utterance is internally related to the proactive feature. Take for instance the health visitor's turn from the interview in Linell's chapter (Chapter 7, p. 160):

H: That's very good. That's very good. And did he lose on his birthweight at all while you were in hospital or. . .

The health visitor's contribution is *retroactive*, i.e. it is a response to the mother, confirming that the health visitor has understood and confirmed the mother's previous turn about her baby's birthweight. However, the health visitor's turn is also *proactive*, i.e. it initiates further exploration of the discussed subject matter by asking whether the baby has lost any weight while in hospital, and thus expands on what has already been mutually established between the health visitor and the mother. In this particular case the *response* to the mother, i.e. 'That's very good. That's very good', and the *initiative*, i.e. 'And did he lose on his birthweight at all while you were in hospital or. . .', are both clearly identifiable parts in the health visitor's turn.

In reality, though, many dialogical turns may only be responses while others may only be initiatives. For example, a turn may be only a brief response, e.g. 'yes' or 'no'. Moreover, in many cases we cannot simply say: 'these words or this phrase amount to the retroactive part and this phrase amounts to the proactive part.' Let us consider, for example, a fragment from Maeterlinck's drama *Intérieur* (Maeterlinck, 1939, p. 181). In this fragment the participants' intersubjective understanding is so great that their dialogue appears to be monologized, with one turn simply elaborating upon the previous one in such a way that their contributions can, imaginably, be made by one person only, rather than by two individuals (Mukařovský, 1940/1977). In the context of my argument, this fragment serves the purpose of showing that in this particular case one cannot, meaningfully, physically separate the retroactive and proactive parts of the participants' turns. The context of the fragment is a conversation between two people, a Stranger and an Old Man. They stand outside the house and watch a family inside through a window:

The Stranger: See, they are smiling in the silence of the room. . .
The Old Man: They are not at all anxious – they did not expect her this evening.

> *The Stranger:* They sit motionless and smiling. But see, the
> father puts his finger to his lips. . .
> *The Old Man:* He points to the child asleep on its mother's
> breast. . .
> *The Stranger:* She dares not raise her head for fear of disturbing
> it. . .
> *The Old Man:* They are not sewing anymore. There is a dead
> silence. . .

In this dialogue each turn as a whole is a response to the previous turn. Yet simultaneously it is, as a whole, an initiative of new content and new images. Since the turn is both an initiative and response *as a whole*, it would be impossible to subdivide it physically into a response-part and an initiative-part. Yet, *conceptually*, it is meaningful to talk in terms of such a subdivision. Thus while in some cases conceptual and physical subdivision into a response-part and an initiative-part may coincide, this is not so in other cases and therefore the two kinds of analysis should not be confused with one another.

A three-step unit as a minimum interaction

The cases we have just discussed focus on single turns as three-step units of analysis in a dialogue. However, one can also take as a starting-point a situation that fulfils the minimum conditions for interaction between two interlocutors to occur. A classic example of this situation is Mead's 'conversation of gestures', in which the minimum unit involves a speaker A, a second speaker B, and speaker A again. Speaker A initiates the interaction, speaker B responds to A and speaker A completes the minimum interactive triad by responding to B's response to his or her own original initiative.

$$A_1 \text{ (step 1)} \qquad B_1 \text{ (step 2)}$$
$$A_2 \text{ (step 3)}$$

Step 3 could be A's expressed attitude with regard to steps 1 and 2, or some other way by which the interaction between steps 1 and 2 is manifested. Step 3, while completing one minimum interaction process, may also serve as step 1 of the next triad in the dialogical process (see Figure 1).

However, let us imagine that A and B pass each other in the street and all they say is:

A: Hi
B: Hi

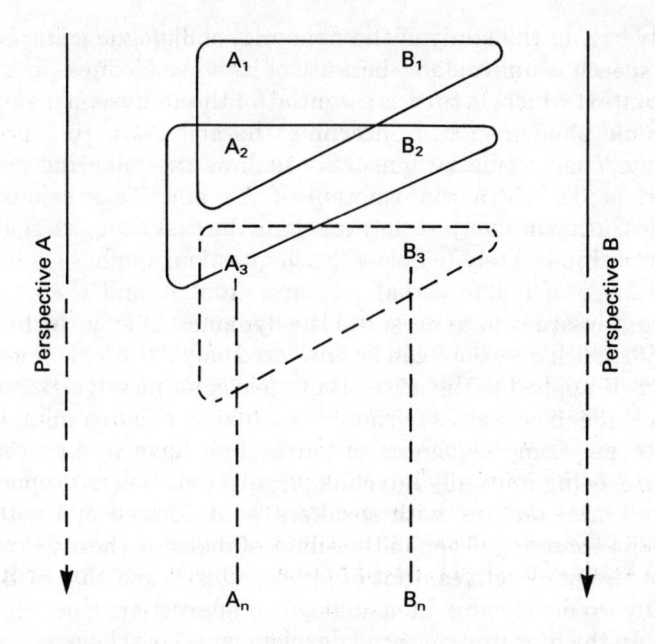

Figure 1 A three-step process and co-development of the perspectives of A and B

One might be tempted to argue that since in this case only two turns have taken place, there are exceptions to the claim that all dialogical interaction is based on three steps. It could be argued that any attempt to impose an imagined third step upon the simple greeting–greeting pair in order to accommodate it in the framework of three-step processes is pushing matters too far. I would claim, however, that such an argument would be yet another attempt to substitute an analysis based on physical units for a conceptual three-step analysis. According to the logic of internal relations, mutually interacting phenomena must give rise to a third phenomenon for the process to be completed. In the case of the greeting–greeting pair, even if the third step is not manifested externally by speech, its existence should be presupposed for the act of communication to be completed. A's and B's exchange of 'Hi' is completed only if A becomes aware of B's 'Hi' and responds to it, at least mentally. For example, A may reflect on the exchange of 'Hi' examining the appropriateness of B's 'Hi' as a response to his or her own 'Hi', the tone of voice, or the expression of 'Hi' against the possibility of silence, and so on. While I accept that for certain kinds of analysis of speech one may not wish to go beyond what the speakers actually say, in the study of the dynamics of dialogue going beyond actual speech is unavoidable because of its embeddedness in a wider social context which, in turn, is essential for the analysis of dialogue as a dynamic phenomenon. Concerning the above greeting–greeting exchange, there could be questions such as the following for A to answer: is B's 'Hi' a confirmation of A's and B's previous relationships? Alternatively, if they meet for the first time, what quality of relationship is likely to follow? Such questions might be answered on the basis of a non-verbal response from A and they may be important in order to understand the dynamics of even such a brief exchange. Such questions can be answered only if the logic of internal relations is applied to the analysis of the communicative exchange.

A dialogue, however, is normally much longer than a minimum of three turns. Long sequences of turns may have a very complex structure, being mutually interlinked, with some topics dropped and restarted later on, and with speakers' goals shifted and with new intentions occurring. Even in the simplest dialogue there are always at least two perspectives, that of interlocutor A and that of B, both mutually co-developing in a dialogical interaction (see Figure 1 above). In the literature of social developmental psychology, mutuality and synchronization of gestures, carefully monitored by the participants in dialogue, have been described by a number of researchers (e.g. Brazelton, Koslowski and Main, 1974; Schaffer, 1979). Indeed, the detailed sequential analyses carried out by these researchers show the importance, for effective communication between the child and his or her caretaker, of the synchronization of gestures between the participants. Whilst such dialogues are always *reciprocal*, in the sense that both interlocutors contribute to its dynamics and their interaction is always a *co-development* of their individual perspectives, such co-development is rarely *symmetrical* (Luckmann, this volume, Chapter 2; Linell, this volume, Chapter 7). Asymmetricity in the co-development of the interlocutors' perspectives is due to various kinds of dominance and power relationships between the interlocutors and to their resulting interdependencies.

A three-step unit cutting across a turn

In all the examples of the analysis of dialogues discussed so far the turns have been treated as homogeneous units in the sense that their internal characteristics have not been specifically considered. Thus a turn in Linell, Gustavsson and Juvonen's (1988) analysis is taken as a whole so that it can be placed in one of eighteen categories in their system for the analysis of interactional dominance. In the Meadian type of interaction, again, it is taken for granted that a turn is homogeneous: one speaker makes a contribution and the other responds, e.g. corroborates, disputes or disregards the other's contribution. In this kind of analysis, in which dialogical turns are considered to be homogeneous units with clearly defined boundaries, the physical and conceptual units of analysis often appear to coincide. Analysis based on the view that turns are homogeneous may, therefore, lead to results that implicitly reinforce the view that physical subdivision into turns is the most natural point of departure in the analysis of dialogues. However, such a view does not hold once we focus attention on the internal characteristics of a turn.

In his analysis of dramatic dialogue Mukařovský (1940/1977) shows that subdivision of a dialogue into turns is secondary to what he he calls the *dialogical quality of speech*. He claims that the dialogical quality of speech is not concentrated at the boundaries between turns, but that it uniformly saturates the entire speech (*ibid.*, p. 108). By dialogical quality Mukařovský means the internal argumentative nature of a turn that is responsible for its dramatic impact on the audience. For example, in one part of a turn the speaker may argue, dispute or question what he or she has conveyed in the other part of the same turn. Discussing Burian's dramatization of the short story by Victor Dyk, 'The Pied Piper of Hamelin', Mukařovský draws attention to semantic reversals within single turns that are calculated to surprise the other interlocutor and to ignore the expected dialogical conventions of local coherence (see Foppa, this volume, Chapter 8) and adopted rules of topic progression and maintenance (see Bergman, this volume, Chapter 9). Consider the following extract from Burian's dramatization:

> *Agnes* (with laughter): Quite a large rat appeared at Katherine's wedding. The groom was as white as a sheet, and Katherine fell into a swoon.
> *Pied Piper*: Any trifle can spoil people's appetite. Are you preparing for a wedding or a christening?

In this extract the speaker, Pied Piper, starts continuing on Agnes's topic. However, in the following utterance he makes a sudden shift, asking Agnes, an unmarried young woman, quite unexpectedly, whether she is preparing for a wedding or for a christening. Such sudden shifts of topics are generally marked by the speaker's intonation, facial expressions, accompanying gestures and by other dialogical qualities that significantly contribute to the dramatic impact of a dialogue. As Mukařovský (1940/1977, p. 109) remarked, the more dramatic the dialogue the more saturated it will be with semantic reversals, regardless of the boundaries of the turns.

Semantic reversals are important communicative strategies in dialogues between professionals and clients. For example, in a counselling interview between a doctor and a patient suffering from AIDS the doctor may, within a single utterance or a turn, switch from using a semantically less loaded term such as 'illness' to a semantically loaded term such as 'AIDS'. Such a semantic reversal may manifest a change in the implicit contract between doctor and patient concerning the way the patient's situation is handled. The turning point in the manner of the doctor may mean a proposal, for the patient, to accept the diagnosis of the illness that he or she has been trying, until now, to deny. In view of such a diagnosis it may mean that certain plans for the patient's future must be reconsidered; and so on. More generally, words and speech actions have diagnoses and prognoses built into their meaning. It is the speaker's privilege to choose how to describe things in order semantically to convert the status quo: to signal changes in interpersonal relations, to diagnose events, to make prognoses about them and to convey his or her changed feelings. It is, of course, up to the listener to dispute, reject or accept the speaker's choice of terms. Thus whether a killing of a human being is called manslaughter, assassination or murder is not just a substitution of one term by the other but an important dialogical device.

These cases show that an analysis of dialogue or its parts into three-step units may be independent of turns and may actually cut across them. If the problem to be explored concerns, say, the development or maintenance of the topic, semantic reversals *within* a turn may become conceptual and possibly physical boundaries defining steps of the analytical unit. Focusing on reversals within turns, the researcher may systematically explore attempts of the speakers to dominate, semantically, the other participants. Moreover, and as Bakhtin (1981) has shown, a dialogue fulfils several purposes at the same time. In the course of his discussion of heteroglossia or multivoicedness, Bakhtin draws attention to the problem as to how, in mutual competition with each other, different contexts and multiple meanings of single words strive to achieve some unity within a single dialogue.

Implications of the conception of three-step processes

The fact that the analysis of a dialogue into three-step units is primarily conceptual and only secondarily physical has important methodological implications. It is the problem to be explored that leads the researcher to determine the level at which the three-step units are defined, i.e. whether at the level of utterances, turns, minimal interactions, semantic reversals, topics or any other dialogical parts. Consequently, such problem-specific three-step units cannot be applied, without consideration that may involve redefinition of the unit or other changes within the unit, to the solution of a problem for which the three-step unit was not intended in the first place. For example, if the research problem is to investigate interactional dominance in dyads in terms of initiative–response (Linell, this volume, Chapter 7), a three-step process defined in terms of this particular problem cannot be used to explore, say, semantic dominance or even interactional dominance in groups because the category system in question can only be used for the solution of a particular kind of problem. While this statement may appear trivial, the transport of a technique or a method from one kind of problem to another is not unusual in psychology. An inexperienced and enthusiastic researcher often perceives a technique as a ready-made tool for exploring problems of his or her own, no matter what they are. If subsequently the tool fails to answer the researchers' question it is criticized as unsatisfactory while the researchers totally ignore the fact that the technique was not designed to examine their kind of problem.

The claim that three-step units are problem-driven and problem-specific can be compared with the claim, sometimes made by conversation analysts, that their approach is *data-driven* (Sacks, 1984). According to the data-driven approach the researcher should have no preconceived ideas about the data and must not impose any theory upon them. This approach of analysis seems to provide these researchers with a heuristic framework within which certain kinds of sequential or instantial characteristics of dialogue can be identified and described. Whether, however, it is possible to describe something without any pre-formed theory is a different question (cf. Kuhn, 1962).

In the present discussion a number of problems have remained implicit and many questions unanswered. For example, three-step processes are assumed to involve both linguistic and extra-linguistic phenomena and the problems arising from the relationships between them remain to be addressed. Moreover, heteroglossia and the multifunctional nature of speech in dialogues raise different kinds of issues when viewed from the point of view of the speaker and when viewed from the point of view of the listener (Farr and Anderson, 1983). The functions (or multifunctions) of particular dialogical signs may be vastly divergent for the addresser and addressee, each of whom may be pursuing his or her own intentions and purposes. Bakhtin analysed the novel as a multiform phenomenon and one can apply his analysis equally well to dialogical face-to-face interactions. One can say that in a dialogue, just as in a novel, 'the investigator is confronted with several heterogeneous stylistic unities, often located on different linguistic levels and subject to different stylistic controls' (Bakhtin, 1981, p. 261). How are speakers' choices of linguistic signs realized under such complex conditions? What are the limits of such choices? Such questions have yet to be answered.

References

Atkinson, M. and Heritage, J. (eds) (1984), *Structures of Social Action*, Cambridge: Cambridge University Press.
Bakhtin, M. M. (1981), *The Dialogic Imagination: Four essays by M. M. Bakhtin*, M. Holquist (ed.), trans. C. Emerson and M. Holquist, Austin: University of Texas Press.
Brazelton, T. B., Koslowski, B. and Main, M. (1974), 'The origins of reciprocity: The early mother–infant interaction', in M. Lewis and L. A. Rosenblum (eds), *The Effect of the Infant on its Caregiver*, London and New York: Wiley.
Drew, P. (1990), 'Strategies in the contest between lawyer and witness, cross-examination', in J. Levi and A. Walker (eds), *Language in the Judicial Process*, New York and London: Plenum.
Farr, R. M. and Anderson, A. (1983), 'Beyond actor/observer differences in perspective: extensions and applications', in M. Hewstone (ed.), *Attribution Theory: Social and functional extensions*, Oxford: Blackwell.
Fichte, J. G. (1794/1970), *Grundlage der gesammten Wissenschaftslehre*, Leipzig: Gabler; 1970 Hamburg: Meiner.
Gibson, J. J. (1979), *The Ecological Approach to Visual Perception*, Boston: Houghton-Mifflin.
Harris, E. E. (1983), *An Interpretation of the Logic of Hegel*, Lanham and New York: University Press of America.
Hegel, G. W. F. (1812–16), *Science of Logic*, trans. A. V. Miller, London and New York: George Allen & Unwin, 1969; New York: Humanities Press, 1976.
Herbst, D. (1987a), 'Co-genetic logic. The eight process networks', Oslo, doc. 1/87 from Work Research Institutes.
Herbst, D. (1987b), 'Man and Machine. The different nature of contextual and modular functioning', Oslo, doc. 21/87 from Work Research Institutes.
Humboldt, W. von (1836/1971), *Linguistic Variability and Intellectual Development*, trans. G. C. Buck and F. A. Raven, Coral Gables: University of Miami Press, 1971,
Jefferson, G. (1989), 'List-construction as a task and resource', in J. Psathas (ed.), *Interactional Competence*, New York: Irvington.
Karcevskij, S. (1929/1982), 'Du dualisme asymetrique du signe linguistique', *Travaux du Cercle Linguistique de Prague*, 1, 88–92. Reprinted as 'The asymmetric dualism of the linguistic sign', in P. Steiner (ed.), *The Prague*

School: Selected writings, 1919–46, Austin: University of Texas Press, 1982.
Kreckel, M. (1981), *Communicative Acts and Shared Knowledge in Natural Discourse*, London and New York: Academic Press.
Kuhn, T. S. (1962), *The Structure of Scientific Revolutions*, International Encyclopedia of Unified Science, ed. O. Neurath, vol. II, no. 2, Chicago: University of Chicago Press.
Labov, W. and Fanshel, D. (1977), *Therapeutic Discourse: Psychotherapy as conversation*, New York: Academic Press.
Levinson, S. C. (1981), 'The essential inadequacies of speech act models of dialogue', in H. Parret, M. Sbisa and J. Verschuesen (eds), *Possibilities and Limitations of Pragmatics*, Proceedings of the Conference on Pragmatics at Urbino, July 8–14 1979, Amsterdam: Benjamins.
Linell, P., Gustavsson, L. and Juvonen, P. (1988), 'Interactional dominance in dyadic communication: A presentation of initiative–response analysis', *Linguistics*, 26, 415–42.
Maeterlinck, M. (1939), *Morceaux choisis*, Paris: Nelson.
Markovà, I. (1987), 'On the interaction of opposites in pschological processes', *Journal for the Theory of Social Behaviour*, 17, 279–99.
Mead, G. H. (1927/1982), '1927 class lectures in social psychology', in D. L. Miller (ed.) (1982), *The Individual and the Social Self*, Chicago and London: The University of Chicago Press.
Mukařovský, J. (1940/1977), 'O jazyce básnickem', *Slovo a Slovesnost*, 6, 113–45. Reprinted as 'On poetic language', in J. Burbank and P. Steiner (eds), *The Word and Verbal Art*, New Haven and London: Yale University Press, 1977.
Pomerantz, A. M. (1984), 'Pursuing a response', in J. Maxwell Atkinson and J. Heritage (eds), *Structures of Social Action*, Cambridge and London: Cambridge University Press.
Rommetveit, R. (1974), *On Message Structure*, New York and London: Wiley.
Sacks, H. (1984), 'Notes on methodology', in J. M. Atkinson and J. Heritage (eds), *Structures of Social Action*, Cambridge: Cambridge University Press; Paris: Editions de la Maison des Sciences de l'Homme.
Saussure, F. (1916/1960), *Cours de Linguistique Générale*, Paris: Payot, trans. W. Baskin, *Course in General Linguistics*, London: Peter Owen, 1960.
Schaffer, H. R. (1979), 'Acquiring the concept of the dialogue', in M. H. Bornstein and W. Kessen (eds), *Psychological Development from Infancy*, Hillsdale, N.J.: Lawrence Erlbaum Associates.
Schegloff, E. A. (1979), 'Repair after next turn', Paper presented at the Social Science Research Council/British Sociological Association Conference on Practical Reasoning and Discourse Processes, St Hugh's College, Oxford.
Schegloff, E. A. (1984), 'On some questions and ambiguities in conversation', in J. Maxwell Atkinson and J. Heritage (eds), *Structures of Social Action*, Cambridge and London: Cambridge University Press.
Schegloff, E. A. and Sacks, H. (1973), 'Opening up closings', *Semiotica*, 7, 289–327.
Searle, J. R. (1969), *On Speech Acts*, Cambridge: Cambridge University Press.
Sinclair, J. and Coulthard, M. (1975), *Towards an Analysis of Discourse*, London: Oxford University Press.

Spencer-Brown, L. (1969), *Laws of Form*, London: George Allen & Unwin.
Tynjanov, J. and Jakobson, R. (1928/1972), 'Problemy izucenija literatury i jazyka', *Novyj Lef*, 12, 36–7. Reprinted in R. T. de George and F. M. de George, *The Structuralists*, Garden City: Doubleday, 1972.
Vološinov, V. N. (1973), *Marxism and the Philosophy of Language*, trans. L. Metajka and I. R. Titunik, New York and London: Seminar Press.
Wiemann, J. M. (1985), 'Interpersonal control and regulation in conversation', in R. L. Street, jr and J. N. Cappella (eds), *Sequence and Pattern in Communicative Behaviour*, London: Edward Arnold.

7 | The power of dialogue dynamics

Per Linell
Department of Communication Studies
University of Linköping

Introduction

This chapter is intended as a contribution to the theory of dialogue, especially as regards the origin and nature of various kinds of *asymmetries* in dialogues embedded in the contexts of social practices of different levels. In the most local context, different options are open to speakers when responding to prior utterances and when initiating new topics and new obligations, and asymmetries are identified on an utterance-to-utterance basis. Thus the power of dialogue dynamics, seen as the *interplay of participants' initiatives and responses*, quite apart from the discourse itself, generates a web of social relations, commitments and responsibilities, and possibly also shared knowledge, attitudes and perspectives. Over and across the sequences of initiatives and responses there emerge patterns of symmetry versus asymmetry (dominance). Such emergent patterns can also be understood partly as reproductions of culturally established and institutionally congealed provisions and constraints on communicative activities.

Data from different sorts of social situations are referred to in this chapter, and some aspects of a theory of dialogue participation structure are conjectured. It is maintained that to focus on asymmetries in dialogue is theoretically and empirically well founded; such

---

This study was financed by a grant awarded to Karin Aronsson and Per Linell by the Bank of Sweden Tercentenary Foundation (RJ 83/137). I wish to thank my collaborators and in particular Karin Aronsson for their help and comments.

asymmetries epitomize some of the most fundamental properties of human interaction.

The social construction of dialogue

There seems to be an increasing consensus among scholars that we must understand social relations, cultural values and cognitive structures as socially produced and reproduced, as socially distributed and organized, as maintained, negotiated, adjusted and established in interaction between individuals who find themselves in social contexts and belonging to cultural traditions. Meanings and rationalities are socially (re-)produced and organized because they are products of interaction between people in social encounters and as such they are subject to social and physical boundary conditions. Meanings (frames and concepts, typifications, folk theories as well as professional knowledge) are socially shared sense-makings of the world. However, in a complex, diversified society people will have partially divergent experiences, and thus knowledge, values and attitudes will be differentially distributed, i.e. they are 'partially shared and only fragmentarily known' in a pluralistic world (Rommetveit, 1983). It is therefore necessary to have a look at the reproduction of intersubjectivity in a cultural and historical perspective (Vygotsky; Bakhtin; Marková, this volume, Introduction).

Meanings are not entirely constructed *ab novo* in interaction; they belong to a cultural capital inherited and reinvested by new actors all the time. Communicative activities are interactionally constructed and managed, historically sedimented and institutionally congealed (Berger and Luckmann, 1967). In others words, microcontexts cannot be understood without some concept of macroframes (ethnographic and organizational contexts) (Cicourel, 1981). Yet, in this chapter I will approach the problems from the microcontext end of the scale, and we will only catch a few glimpses of the wider cultural ecologies involved.

This is not the place to argue for social constructivism (see e.g. Schutz, 1967, and later Berger and Luckmann, 1967; Heritage, 1984; Rommetveit, 1987). Nor is there space to explore the complexity of the dialectical relations, the interdependence, between key notions like meaning and context, thought and communication, expression and content, construction and tradition. I will simply assume that meaning is both context-dependent and an accomplishment and product of social (contextualized) practices, that thought is at the same time presupposed, processed and produced in inter- and intra-individual communication, that differences of form (expression) usually entail differences in content and vice versa, and that there is a dialogical relation (Bakhtin, 1986) in communicative acts between what is created and produced and what is given, fixed, conventional and often taken for granted. On all these issues (and others that could be added), fundamental arguments for a Hegelian view (rather than the usual Cartesian view) have been advanced (Marková, 1982).

Dialogue, like social interaction in general, is dynamic in nature. The dynamics of dialogue may be said to reside in the fluctuating interdependencies between dialogue partners, and in the progression of actor-produced dyadic states, where actors are constantly dependent on perceptions and interpretations of each other's actions. Communicative acts, e.g. conversational contributions, are always both context-dependent and context-renewing (where 'context' may be understood as the local dialogue context (co-text) but also as a more comprehensive situational frame). To use a terminology I will return to later on, interactants both 'respond' to (their perceptions of) the contextual conditions, expectations and obligations at hand, and also 'initiate' new contextual conditions by saying and doing things. Another dynamic aspect of dialogue is the fact that dialogue is socially, or collectively, constructed and managed in a situational and cultural context. Conversation as an interactional achievement involves the co-construction of both expression and content (interpretation). 'Speaking together' involves the mutual consideration of each other's presumed meanings, intentions and presuppositions leading to at least partially shared understandings.

The analysis of dialogue must therefore concern the relations between at least *three* complexes: *utterance* (or conversational contribution), *understanding* and *context* (Fillmore, 1985). It is not a dual relation between form (utterance) and content as many linguists and semioticians in the past would have it. The intrinsic relationships between our three poles can be expressed in several ways:

1. You understand an utterance by relating it to the context (both local contexts and global frames), i.e. by giving it meaning within a sufficiently coherent (though perhaps fragmentary) network of knowledge.
2. You display (part of) your understanding of contexts by uttering something specific at any given moment in the interaction.
3. You construct or renew the context by producing and/or understanding the utterance.

I am thus deeply opposed to the view of communication as a transportation of fixed meanings (the conduit metaphor of communication in Reddy, 1979) and to the conception of dialogue as a fixed, static text with an intrinsic meaning (Vološinov, 1973; Rommetveit, 1974, 1983, 1988b; Linell, 1982). Dialogue is the locus for the dynamic construction and reconstruction of meaning. Through this process, dialogue expresses, reflects and determines social relations and culture-specific rationalities.

The dialogical interplay of initiatives and responses

Dialogue[1] is a suitable locus for studies of power and dynamics on a scale from the most local contexts — sequences of adjacent dialogue contributions — up to situations and subcultures. I will follow this path in this chapter, starting with the most local contexts.

At the microlevel we can study the local dynamics of speaker–addressee relations on a turn-by-turn basis. Here we see the unfolding joint discourse as produced by context-determined and context-determining moves (conversational contributions). We will call these aspects of utterances *responses* and *initiatives*, respectively. In principle, every conversational contribution (utterance) exhibits both responsive and initiatory features. As Heritage (1987, p. 264) puts it, 'Each social action is a recognizable commentary on, and intervention in, the setting of activity in which it occurs.' Heritage (1984, 1987) firmly belongs in the ethnomethodological 'Conversation Analysis' (CA) tradition. One of the reasons that CA insists on the study of sequential organization in dialogue, rather than focusing on individual speech acts, is precisely because of the insight that an essential property of conversational contributions resides in their context-shaped and context-renewing (i.e. responsive and initiatory) nature. For mainly methodological reasons, CA studies these interrelations solely in terms of their manifestations in the flow of discourse itself.

The Russian tradition of semiotics (Bakhtin, Vološinov) is very different in this respect, in that it relates discourse to a much wider context involving culture and history too. Nevertheless, Bakhtin also regarded the Janus-like response-and-initiative nature of the utterance as the essence of the 'dialogical principle' (Todorov, 1984). A dialogue must be understood as a sequence of interlocking utterances. Wertsch notes that Bakhtin's concept of dialogicality is:

> grounded in the observation that 'any utterance is a link in the chain of speech communication' [Bakhtin] 1986, p. 84. Associated

with this the claim that every utterance responds in some way to previous utterances and anticipates the responses of other, succeeding ones. (Wertsch, 1987, p. 7)

Every utterance has a history in the discourse and an embeddedness in situation and culture, and it also projects possible continuations, more or less likely next-utterances. Marková (this volume, Chapter 6) expresses the same idea when she proposes that 'words and speech actions have diagnoses and prognoses built into their meanings' (p. 140). In my view, both ethnomethodology and Russian social psychology have made major contributions to the conceptual foundations of dialogue theory.

Leaving traditions aside for a moment, let us look at a few aspects of the power of dialogue dynamics. I will start with a rather trivial piece of conversation, taken from a casual exchange between two strangers who meet at a recreation centre out of town. Some utterances are exchanged about running at a nearby jogging track.[2]

I
1. *A*: How long does it take to run the 10 kilometre track?
2. *B*: Up to an hour. That's what it usually takes.
3. *A*: I see. [pause] Six minutes per kilometre.
4. *B*: Yes, but the kilometres are not really equally long on that track.
5. *A*: Oh, well, the ground varies like that?
6. *B*: Yes, that too, but then the distances aren't equally long between the markings [i.e. kilometre markings].

In this extract, A starts by asking a question, which of course amounts to a conversational initiative; B is put under the obligation when continuing the dialogue to keep to the condition that he provide a relevant answer (or, at least, by giving some reason why he could not do so). In this case, he does give an answer, though hardly more than a minimal answer. In other words, B does not take any independent initiative of his own. This leaves A with an opportunity, even an implicit responsibility, to accept and give some credit to B for his response. A does this ('I see'), but he also uses his turn to add a reflection, which, at the same time, may be said to display A's understanding of B's response. It is therefore (possibly) also an explanation for why he asked the question in 1 in the first place. Now B, in 4, reacts to A's interpretation in 3, carrying on the dialogue by taking a new, though topically relevant, initiative. A, in 5, does not appear to be quite sure how to understand B's remark, and accordingly, his response to 4 involves a new initiative, requesting more information. B gives this, thus using his turn to explain what he meant (or may have meant) by his preceding remark (4). In this way, the dialogue is collectively brought forward by the interlocutors' responding to each other and taking new initiatives – in Heritage's terms (see above), by commenting on the preceding contributions and making new interventions. At the same time, the actors are seen to display their unfolding understanding of the joint discourse on a moment-to-moment basis. Incidentally, we may note that understanding is not something which is necessarily 'there' before verbalization. Thus, to an observer it is not evident that B, when uttering 4, was already aware that what he meant by it was precisely what, just a few moments later, he explained as 6. (As a matter of fact, I happen to know that B was *not* fully aware of it, since I was B in this example!) Understanding develops in and through the dialogue itself. In Schegloff's (1982, p. 75) words:

> The discourse should be treated as an achievement; that involves treating the discourse as something 'produced' over time, incrementally accomplished, rather than born naturally whole out of the speaker's forehead, the delivery of a cognitive plan.

As we can see, we can study the dynamic relations between utterance, meaning and context at work on a turn-to-turn basis. Each contribution or turn is dependent on the preceding turn(s), but it also partially determines the conditions for relevant next turns. Many utterances must be seen as multifunctional and ambiguous. There is an inherent 'incompleteness' in a linguistic expression in that it does not 'carry with it' its meaning. Rather, meaning is a locally produced accomplishment and interactants use their turns in talking to display their understanding of the preceding utterances in their context. In this way interpretation, whether exposed in actual utterances or merely intra-individual, largely builds up coherence in discourse (Hopper, 1983). This also implies that there is a continuous interplay between the production and understanding aspects of communicative activities. In fact, understanding is not simply displayed in discourse; it is (at least to some extent) *created* (achieved) through the verbalization act itself. In Rommetveit's terms (1988a), 'making sense of' something and 'bringing it into language' are two aspects of the same complex process (also Rommetveit, this volume, Chapter 4).

There is an inherent power in dialogue to generate further dialogue: understanding of previous contributions is displayed in responses, expansions and new initiatives, and utterances project new utterances to come. With Maturana and Varela (1987), who compare dialogue to a living organism, we might think of this ability as a 'self-reproducing (self-organizing) principle' in dialogue. (It seems evident, however, that a theory of autopoietic systems, regarding them as independent of external forces (Maturana and Varela, 1980) is not sufficient to account for the mutually constitutive nature of dialogue contributions and contexts (Rommetveit, this volume, Chapter 4).) So far, I have used the term 'power' in a somewhat loose, perhaps partly metaphorical sense. However, since initiatives and responses have to do with controlling versus being controlled, there is also a sense in which *social power* is exercised within the social encounter, at a microlevel. The point, then, is to see this 'micropower' as a very elementary form of power.

Wrong (1968, p. 673) notes that 'asymmetry exists in each individual act–response sequence'. The speaker has a certain privilege in being able to take initiatives and display his or her own understanding. However, there is a continuous reciprocity of influence, since 'the actors continually alternate the roles of power holder and power subject in the total course of their interaction' (*ibid.*, p. 673). Yet dialogues and situations characteristically differ in the global effects of these role alternations. Quite often, one party comes out as dominant – in one or several dimensions (see pages 155–7). For example, asking questions is a matter of trying to condition the other's contributions more or less strongly, whereas simply answering questions may amount to little more than just complying with the other's conditions. There are many ways of varying the strength of conversational contributions. It is therefore often quite instructive to study how and by whom the dialogue is driven forward in different situations.

Our next example is taken from a radio phone-in on the Swedish network (*Ring så spelar vi* with Hasse Tellemar), in which listeners are invited to phone the programme presenter, and the ensuing conversations are broadcast. Basically, presenter and caller chat for a while about everyday matters. The excerpt below is taken from this phase (though there are also other phases in the conversation, such as the caller's being asked a quiz question).

II

P = programme presenter; *C* = middle-aged female caller

1. *P*: What more shall we say about this day? The sun is shining here at the moment
2. *C*: Yes, but it isn't here
3. *P*: It will

4. *C*: It's coming, 'cause there's a dog exhibition here at Sjöhagen this weekend, and then we'll need some sun...
5. *P*: Yes, and are you going there with your doggie?
6. *C*: No, you see, I too... 've taken him away (a dialectal euphemism for 'kill' is used), we talked about that in May, you an' I
7. *P*: *Did* we?
8. *C*: Yes
9. *P*: You know, when you said Sandbäck (the caller's name), it occurred to me then that this lady had called before
10. *C*: Yes
11. *P*: And we had a talk in May, you say
12. *C*: Yes, on the national day of Norway
13. *P*: The seventeenth of May
14. *C*: Yes
15. *P*: Mm, OK
16. *C*: Then we had taken him away three days earlier
17. *P*: I see
18. *C*: So today we have recovered reasonably well
19. *P*: Well, it takes some time
20. *C*: It will take a long time, as long as one doesn't get hold of anything new either...

Excerpt II is a piece of reasonably balanced conversation with both parties taking a number of initiatives, interspersed with turns which are more like minimal responses. The caller brings in a couple of topics of her own, which is hardly surprising, given that these phone-in programmes tend to zoom in on the caller's life. The presenter contributes to the progression of the dialogue – after all, it is his responsibility that something gets said – but his methods consist in rather phatically oriented invitations (e.g. 1; 9; 11). For comparison, look at excerpt III which is drawn from another, very similar phone-in (*Upp till tretton* with Ulf Elfving), the relevant difference being that callers on this programme are always children of at most 13 years of age. (Another difference is that the youngsters have sent in postcards in advance, giving some information about themselves, and actually, *they* are called up by the radio network employees, although this part is not broadcast.) The conversations typically take on a different character, with the programme presenter asking questions almost all the time. The caller's role is thereby reduced to one of responding to initiatives from the interlocutor, with a few voluntary expansions now and then. The exchange type seems quite typical of a child's conversation with an adult stranger.

III
Excerpt from a conversation with a 10-year-old boy (C)

1. P: Are you interested in being busy working with your hands, can you do woodwork and such things?
2. C: Yes, a little
3. P: Mm, have you ever made a bark boat?
4. C: No
5. P: You haven't, no, but you do other things perhaps
6. C: Yes
7. P: What then?
8. C: Well, now that I have woodwork at school, then I have made some dice and such things, pencil stands and . . .
9. P: I see. How is . . . what's the bird's name, is it . . .
10. C: Kalle
11. P: Kalle, I see, I thought he had some other name. Kalle is it, what kind of bird is it?
12. C: It's a budgy
13. P: That can talk?
14. C: No,
15. P: No, there are just a few budgies that talk, of course. Anyway, he sings?
16. C: Mm
17. P: That's good. (2 sec) And then you have many nice pals in Åsby?
18. C: Yes
19. P: (faintly) 's written here. (louder) Åsby is in the middle of Skåne, more or less, isn't it?
20. C: Yes

It may be that III is fairly extreme in its asymmetry, even given the specific genre to which it belongs. However, most people will recognize the pattern of a benevolent adult who does his or her best with a shy and reticent, maybe even reluctant, child. The adult brings the discourse forward by introducing new topics and topic aspects and by trying to invite contributions from his or her passive interlocutor. Invitations, however, are not enough: the speaker has to ask explicit questions most of the time (soliciting initiatives). The subordinate party in excerpt III does little more than what is minimally required, given his interlocutor's questions. Often, he does not even do this adequately, though the presenter tends to avoid pressing him (but see turn 7, which explicitly treats 6 as insufficient). An important point to observe is that the resulting dialogue is a *collective* product: both parties exert influence over it. It is true that the presenter interactionally dominates his young interlocutor by forcing him to answer rather specific questions, but there is no doubt that the child's passivity also contributes to this pattern – without the presenter's persistent questioning, the dialogue would probably have come to a complete standstill. In other words, it always takes two to produce a dialogue; both parties are intercursively defining conditions for each other's contributions.

To recapitulate, in the progression of dialogue from utterance to utterance (or turn to turn) there is local reciprocity, an 'attunement to the attunement of the other' (Rommetveit, this volume, Chapter 4), embodied in the Janus-like nature of the individual utterance or turn. This is accompanied by a basic asymmetry inherent in the difference between the roles of speaker and addressee. Rommetveit (1987, p. 90) characterizes the dialogical condition as follows:

> the dyadic constellation of speaker's privilege and listener's commitment: the speaker has the privilege of determining what is being referred to and/or meant, whereas the listener is committed to making sense of what is said by temporarily adopting the speaker's perspective on the talked-about state of affairs.

The speaker role is also associated with provisions to govern and control (or let him- or herself be governed and controlled). One might say that further asymmetries may be generated over and above the basic one: there is more to local power than what inheres in the speaker role as such.

There are cases of dialogues developing into symmetrical talk-exchanges: when person A has made a contribution, person B gives a relevant and expanded response to A's utterance, thereby providing further topic resources for the ensuing discourse; then A in his or her turn likewise provides a relevant and expanded response, then B continues in the same way, etc. There are also several ways of generating asymmetries deviating from this symmetric pattern by deploying the dynamics of initiatives-and-responses in specific ways. For example, a speaker can demand or solicit responses rather than just invite them; as we noted earlier, if he or she asks questions, he or she makes answers obligative rather than facultative. On the other hand, a speaker can inhibit further talk on a topic, for example by initiating new topics. Another instance of dominant behaviour is to make meta-communicative comments on the partner's utterances (rather than responding to them topically), or simply to ignore the other's contributions and connect to one's own prior utterances. The

The power of dialogue dynamics 157

latter would lead to a halting and less well co-ordinated dialogue (what Linell, Gustavsson and Juvonen, 1988, have termed 'obliqueness'). These are examples of domineering behaviour. The subordinate party's weapon, unless he or she wants to counter-attack by attempting moves similar to the ones just mentioned, is to respond minimally or to refuse to respond. This kind of resistant behaviour will also have a decisive influence on the dialogue, as excerpt III demonstrated.

Initiatives and responses are local events. Many contributions of similar kinds, however, may add up to aggregated patterns emerging over sequences of utterances. For example, if one party keeps asking questions and his or her partner can do nothing but give answers on the conditions set up by the questions, we will get a summative pattern of interactional dominance for the former speaker. Linell, Gustavsson and Juvonen (1988) have explored the idea of computing various quantitative measures of dominance and coherence in dialogue by looking at properties of sequences. As will be conjectured below (see pages 166–70), such measures can be used in diagnosing social situations. First, however, we need to look a little closer at some kinds of dominance in dialogue.

Dimensions of dominance

Although some of my prior remarks might invite a discussion of the major sociological issues of power and exchange, it is not possible to give them anything like adequate treatment in this context. My objective is rather different: I propose a study of some local and global properties of dialogue. In particular, I want to discuss some aspects of dominance and asymmetries in dialogue. I shall then use the term 'dominance' to refer to various more or less visible (manifest) dimensions or structures in dialogue and discourse. 'Power' can arguably be conceived of as more abstract than dominance and as involving an invisible (latent) macrostructure.[3] Dimensions of dominance in dialogue can be identified without any *specific* a priori assumptions of social order and social power; instead, dialogue analyses *per se* may lead us to a model of the provisions for and constraints on different sorts of social situations and communicative activities (see pages 166–70). These provisions and constraints are, of course, partly imposed or supported from outside, via institutionalized rules and social power relations (e.g. courtroom procedural rules, or norms for and expectations of adult–child interaction). However, they are also reproduced through the particular patterns of situated collaborative action; that is, they can be understood partly as generated 'from within', through the dynamics of the self-organizing principle of dialogue (Luckmann, this volume, Chapter 2).

Dominance in interaction is multidimensional: there are many different ways in which a party can be said to 'dominate', i.e. possess or control the 'territory' to be shared by the communicating parties. The territory, of course, is the jointly attended and produced discourse.[4] Dominance is a property of *sequences* of entire social interactions (dialogues) or of phases within them. (Asymmetries, in my terminology, could also be local.) There are at least four different dimensions involved in dominance in interaction: amount of talk, semantic dominance, interactional dominance and strategic moves.

With respect to the first dimension, the dominant party is simply the one who talks the most (purely quantitative dominance). Semantic (or topic) dominance would apply if one party predominantly introduced and maintained topics and perspectives on topic (see below). Interactional dominance would deal with patterns of asymmetry in terms of initiative–response (IR) structure. The dominant party is the one who makes most initiatory moves (contributions that strongly determine the unfolding local context) and makes relatively fewer weak moves (in which responding aspects prevail). The subordinate party of the interaction, on the other hand, allows his or her contributions to be directed, controlled and/or inhibited by the interlocutor's surrounding moves. Finally, we distinguish strategic moves as a special type of dominance device: you need not talk a lot or make many strong moves, as long as you say a few, strategically really important things.

Interactional dominance is that aspect which will interest us most in this chapter. The reason, as I have already pointed out, is that it nicely ties up with the basic properties of dialogue contributions: their responsive and initiating features. In a series of empirical studies (e.g. Gustavsson, 1988; Linell, Gustavsson and Juvonen, 1988), we have developed a so-called 'initiative–response' (IR) analysis, which is built upon an operationalization of a number of turn types (categories of conversational contributions) in terms of a coding scheme. In this analysis, initiatives are further classified as more or less strong appeals to the interlocutor to respond under given conditions, and responses are categorized with regard to how and to what extent they are in fact determined by the other's initiatives. Such types of dialogue contributions are assigned different interactional strength (or weight) on a six-point ordinal scale, and it thus becomes possible to calculate, among other things, the average interactional strength of each actor's contributions (IR index = median value of interactional strength). We can then also derive a numerical value for the *IR difference* of the dyad as the difference between actors' IR indices. The IR difference we take as an indicator of interactional asymmetry. For example, this difference would be small in a relatively symmetrical relationship such as that between caller and programme presenter in excerpt II (IR difference = 0.21), and large in the correspondingly asymmetrical relationship in excerpt III (IR difference = 2.01) (differences increase with increasing interactional asymmetry).[5]

Unlike most traditional coding schemes for interaction analysis (from Bales, 1950, onwards) which are more or less speech-act based, IR analysis shares some major theoretical assumptions with the traditions referred to above (see pages 148–9). Methodologically, it is of course entirely different; indeed, Conversation Analysis (Atkinson and Heritage, 1984, p. 3) tends to reject coding schemes and quantification entirely as methodological tools in the analysis of dialogue. Similarly, Bakhtinian dialogue theory cannot of course be directly applied in ordinary empirical work, nor can it be specified in terms of a workable category system.[6]

Interactional dominance

With respect to interactional dominance (and domineeringness), we find at least three main types of strong initiatives: *directing* moves, *controlling* moves and *inhibiting* moves. The first category comprises moves by which the speaker tries to force the other to respond under certain conditions. These are questions and directives in traditional terms. Asking questions is a well-known dominant strategy (unless we are faced with submissive questions, by which a party, often a subordinate one, shows deference and respect by suggesting that the other party talk). Of course, questioning can be handled in many ways. One strategy, which leaves little room for the interviewee to expand, is to have a battery of questions which are asked in sequence with no or infrequent comments on the answers received. The short excerpt (IV) below is taken from that phase of a police interrogation in which the police officer goes through a number of fixed questions when filling in a form about the suspect's personal circumstances.

IV
P: Sven Erik Andersson . . . it was Erik you said, wasn't it?
S: Yes
P: (9 sec) 55-07-11 (5 sec) 5386 (civil registration number which P takes from his file) (4 sec) occupation, what do I write there?
S: Officer-of-state

P: What?
S: Officer-of-state
P: Oh yes (13 sec) In which parish are you registered?
S: um . . . St Nicholas
P: OK (7 sec) Married or single?
S: Single

(Police interrogation, No. 10:1; Jönsson, 1988)

The format of many such questions in sequence is almost maximally constraining on possible responses and seldom gives rise to responses (on the part of the questioner) to the answers given. The filling in of blanks on the forms of various institutions is the prototypical case. (It might be the case that such formats become more frequent and even more extreme when routines are computerized.) A rather less domineering way of requesting information from a client is to give some feedback – sometimes second assessments or even second stories (Pomerantz, 1984) – upon receiving answers, before the next question is asked. The following is a short extract from an interview involving a health visitor and a woman who has recently had a baby (example given by courtesy of John Heritage, Heritage and Sefi (forthcoming).

V

H: How much does he weigh?
M: He's $8\frac{1}{2}$ pounds now.
H: Lovely, lovely. Did the midwife weigh him before you were discharged or . . .
M: Yes. He was weighed today.
H: Oh lovely. What was his birthweight?
M: Seven eleven.
H: That's very good. That's very good. And did he lose on his birthweight at all while you were in hospital or . . .
M: Well they didn't weigh him until he was a week old, so I don't really know.
H: Yes, yes. Oh that's super. And is he fairly regular with feeding?

Here too, the interviewer keeps asking questions, but she also uses her turns for providing some feedback, which gives the whole interaction a rather less strict character. Of course, if an interviewer goes beyond this, e.g. by providing more commentaries or perhaps disclosing some things about him- or herself, the interaction would be even less asymmetrical. Questioning strategies of various sorts have been investigated in numerous studies, including some of our own (Adelswärd, Aronsson and Linell, 1988; Linell, Gustavsson and Juvonen, 1988; Aronsson and Sätterlund-Larsson, 1987; Gustavsson, 1988; Adelswärd, 1988; Jönsson, 1988; Adelswärd, Aronsson, Jönsson and Linell, 1987).

Controlling moves are used to evaluate, ratify or disqualify the other's contributions (and the meanings indicated therein). I will give several examples of such moves on pages 161–6 (see also the examples from paediatric consultations to follow).

Interactional dominance may also be exercised by *inhibiting* talk from the other, i.e. by actions depriving him or her of opportunities to participate (lay out his or her version, express his or her wishes etc.). This can be done by explicit framing moves, by which topics or phases are closed. Another, somewhat less explicit way of doing it is to issue 'declarative representatives' (Searle, 1976), i.e. to declare one's own versions or statements as the relevant things to say or as true facts that need not be subjected to further negotiation. As Searle observed, we often 'need an authority to lay down a decision as to what the facts are after the fact-finding procedure has been gone through ... If the judge declares you guilty (on appeal), then for legal purposes you are guilty' (*ibid.*, p. 15). Very often, e.g. in the trials investigated by Adelswärd, Aronsson and Linell (1988), the admission (or denial) of guilt requires a routine-like sequence, in which the defendant's admission (or denial) is restated by the judge. Only then, it seems, is it regarded as a legal fact, as is indicated in the following (slightly simplified) examples.

VI
J: Did you do this?
D: Yes.
J: You admit it (assertive tone).

Or, with an extra confirmation around it.

VII
J: Did you do this?
D: Yes.
J: So you admit it?
D: Yes.
J: OK.

A characteristic type of conversational contribution that is often made by professionals in the course of institutionalized fact-finding procedures is what might be called reformulation (or formulation, according to Heritage and Watson, 1980). This is a rather powerful move by which the speaker both summarizes the gist of, or draws conclusions from, what the interviewee has said and, sometimes somewhat ambiguously, wants him or her to (re-)confirm. Often, the speaker uses his or her reformulation to introduce concepts from his or her (rather than the interviewee's) conceptual framework (on this point, see also pages 163–5 below). This is done by the judge in the following exchange from a Swedish court trial.

VIII
The defendant is accused of tax evasion. He admits not having delivered certain accounts but denies that he intended to withhold tax money.

J: (. . .) Now the prosecutor says that when you did not give in these VAT accounts, it was your intention that taxes should be charged to the company with too low an amount. Is that right?
D: No, it isn't, in that . . ., 'cause those which I got, you see, they went by the county police commissioner so that I . . .
J: Yes, is it so that the circumstances are correct (*D*: Yes) but you deny tax fraud, is that correctly understood?
D: Yes.
       (Trial, No. 23:4; Adelswärd, Aronsson and Linell, 1988)

The relations between different kinds of dominance devices in dyadic communication are further explored and exemplified in Linell, Gustavsson and Juvonen (1988) and Adelswärd, Aronsson and Linell (1988). A partially different type of dominance becomes possible if there are more than two persons present in the conversation. It will then be possible to 'steal' another person's turn or to reformulate or correct the other's contributions. Bruner (1985, p. 31) notes that in adults' conversations with small children, 'the adult serves almost as the vicarious consciousness of the child in the sense of being the only one who knows the goal of the activity the two of them are engaged in.' In a study of paediatric consultations in an allergy clinic, Aronsson and Rundström (1988) observed similar phenomena with parents routinely stepping in as the spokespersons for their children (who in this study were much older, from 5 to 15 years). I will cite a couple of examples from their study, where either the mother simply grabs the child's turn (the doctor is clearly addressing the child) or she comes in right after the child, ratifying and reinforcing what he said and, as it were, explaining what he meant (implying that he could not, or did not get the opportunity to, express it properly himself).

IX
C = a 10-year-old boy

D: And Vilhelm, how are you then?
C: Well, I'm OK
D: You're OK
M: He's got a sore throat when he wakes up during the week, and his nose is blocked up so that he talks through his nose

X
C = another 10-year-old boy

D: You do have sports um of course, don't you?
M: Mm, yeah... twice a week
D: (simultaneously) You can keep up?
C: No, yes well things go well
D: Yes they do
M: That depends of course on what they're doing as well and... if they run running competitions and that kind of thing, then it's not so... then he starts puffing and panting
D: Yeah
M: But otherwise he's with them, I guess, 'cause I talked to his teacher and she says that things are OK, so

Often enough, imputations of dominance can be based upon formal properties of utterances and on small units (single turns) in local contexts. Our examples have been more or less of this kind. However, in order to understand the power dynamics of social situations more fully, we must pay closer attention to meaning and perspectivity and to longer sequences. This we will do in the next section, which will thus also provide us with something like a bridge to (semi-)macrostructures.

Semantic dominance and privileged representations

A substantial portion of the power execution in talk-in interaction consists of constraints on when and for how long parties allow each other to talk (and to think between periods of talk). Directing, inhibiting and framing (i.e. regulative, meta-communicative) moves play an important role in this regard (Schegloff, 1987, pp. 39–40). In institutional contexts of the kinds we have dealt with (court trials, police interviews, doctor consultations, social worker–client interactions etc.), questions have a major function in professionals' discourse. For example, about 80 per cent of all the turns of judges and lawyers are questions (Adelswärd, Aronsson and Linell, 1988). Every time a question is asked, the answerer is put under constraints.[7] It is true that questions vary in coerciveness and that answerers can use their turns to introduce material into discourse other than that which has been strictly asked for, but clients do this to a relatively limited extent. There were more initiatives on the part of clients in the social welfare agency, while there were very few in the court trial and in some phases of the police interviews. Despite the differences, *all* these interviews and interrogations come out as rather asymmetrical when, as in our initiative–response (IR) measures (Linell, Gustavsson and Juvonen, 1988), one aggregates across individual turns and calculates the summative effects of the sustained interactional dominance of professionals.

If an actor is interactionally dominant (has a high IR index, i.e. he takes relatively many strong initiatives), he or she will stand a good chance of enforcing his or her own perspective or rationality on to the joint discourse. Conversely, a subordinate party (with a low IR index, i.e. with many weak responses) will have few opportunities to express his or her own point of view. However, there is no way of uncovering the ways actors use their turns to pursue their topics and perspectives by just looking at IR measures (which simply reflect the interactional functions of turns in their local contexts). Topic perspectives are normally the emergent products of sequences of turns (or of long monological turns). Often, not least in the task-oriented institutional contexts referred to above, sequences of questions (from the professional) are posed in the service of an argumentation, the superordinate goal of which is to provide a certain perspective on the events being described and assessed in the dialogue. Drew (1985) (cf. also Dunstan, 1980) has shown how lawyers in court use the format of coercive questions with (relatively) predictable responses to impose a perspective on things talked about. Here is an example from one of the trials used in our study, where the defence lawyer (DL) uses a series of questions to project an image of the defendant (D) as having been forced into his criminal activities by the threat of physical violence (a mitigating fact, which the defendant was not able to press into the discourse by himself).

XI

The defendant is accused of having rented video boxes and other goods and then sold them to get money for paying back a debt

DL: Did you know or had you rented any such boxes before?
D No, no, not that ...

DL: So it was this person, your creditor, who told you how you should go about doing it, and . . .?
D: Yes, he said so, you know, now you've got your chance and so . . . He knew it, so you have just to step in and rent this, or something like that.
DL: But did you realize that by writing your name on those you um . . .
D: Oh yes, I realized that I would end up here in court, you know, and have to get things straight, you know, but anyway . . .
DL: But you mean that um the alternative was to be struck half dead if you did . . .?
D: Well, half, wholly maybe
DL: And you had no other possibilities to get your money?
D: I called my mum and tried to borrow money, but there was no way there either.

(Trial, No. 41:30–1)

In this case we see a defence lawyer using his privileged position to invoke a perspective on events talked about, and this was in the interest of his client and interactant. In the following examples we see professionals trying to reinterpret things said by defendants in ways that may be alien to the understanding of those defendants. In XII, the defendant (D) is a post-office employee who is accused of fraud. In the excerpt, reference is made to the conditions under which a preceding interview by the police was conducted. The judge (J) is trying to enforce a distinction between 'stressed' and 'pressed', which does not appear to be a clear distinction in the defendant's conceptual world.

XII

DL: Tell us how you experienced the first hearing then.
D: Well, I don't know what to say. Pressed or stressed. Stressed I was mainly I guess because I was in such a hurry. I had a good deal to do at the post office before I could go home. Just to get away as soon as possible.
J: Yes, but pressed or stressed, in this case there is a little difference, isn't there? Pressed, that falls back on the interrogator, doesn't it? And stressed, that is that you are a bit worked up. Which was it?
D: Well, it is difficult to tell now afterwards.
J: (to his secretary) It is difficult to tell if he was pressed or stressed on this . . .

D: Well, stressed I was, that's for sure
J: What?
D: Well, in any case I was stressed
J: But stressed he was in any case. But it is difficult to tell if he was pressed, or what do you mean on this point? Or how do you want it?

The dialogue goes on without the defendant's being able to be more precise about what had happened in the police hearing.

(Trial, No. 8:41–2)

In many social encounters we find two (or more) persons engaged in talk about certain referents or a certain state of affairs (on reference there is often agreement between parties, see pages 155–6 on speaker's responsibility and recipient's commitment). Sometimes, however, the actors disagree on how the state of affairs should be understood and accounted for (what it means or is taken to be an instance of). Often, a superior is in a privileged position (has a privilege of formulation and/or interpretation), as in excerpts XI and XII. Sometimes, parties defend their positions on a more equal basis, as in the abortion trial reported by Danet (1980), where the choice of word (*baby* or *foetus*) is closely tied to the judgement of the whole legal and moral issue involved.

As a further illustration of differences in perspectivity and privileged representations (for this term, see Rorty, 1979), consider an example from Gustavsson (1988, p. 75). It is taken from a lesson in Swedish as a second language. A 12-year-old immigrant boy is talking with his teacher about a text they have read together. The text, drawn from a children's story-book, is about cats. One of them, called Måns, is said to be 'nasty' (Swedish *elak*). The teacher asks her pupil what this word means (one out of many language-based questions being asked in this lesson).

XIII
T: You know it goes like this, the nastiest cat is called Måns, what does that mean?
P: Well he's of the sort that can cheat
T: Mm, but if you are nasty, what are you like then?
P: He's of the sort that doesn't like Pelle (another cat in the story)
T: No but . . . but if . . . if someone is nasty, what is he like then?
P: (4 sec) don't know
T: You don't know, let's look it up and see (*P*: Mm) if we can find an explanation of it

(13 sec)

P: nasty (inaudible sequence)
T: (interrupts) you can almost say someone is unkind, one is evil (P: Yes) if one is nasty, you can write that down, nasty... equals evil, you know what that is, don't you (P: Yes), you are evil towards someone when you are unkind to someone and then you are nasty towards that person

The pupil tries to ground his answers in the text-world that is being talked about. But the teacher intends her question to be taken as pertaining to the decontextualized lexical meaning of the word 'nasty'. Her perspective is an abstract (meta-)linguistic one, founded in the specific (professionalized) activity of language teaching.

In encounters between professionals and lay persons, it happens rather frequently that meanings are negotiated. As we have just noted, this takes the form of discussing how words used (and often introduced) by the layperson should be understood. For example, there is a negotiation of how events in the client's or patient's life should be framed and understood in terms of legal, administrative or medical concepts. Often, and sometimes for good reasons, the final decisions (and agreements) are based on the professional's terms. The social encounter, however, becomes an arena where we witness a clash between different frames, the professional's world of expert knowledge and the layperson's everyday life world. Fragments of the actors' different rationalities and conceptualizations are made visible in the microcontext of dialogue, and, accordingly, voices of the different cultures are heard in actual dialogue. We can see one example in Mishler's (1984) 'voice of medicine' and 'voice of life world' in the medical encounter, another one in Gustavsson's (1988) language lessons where the teacher's frame of lexical meaning collides with the student's sense of meaning based on concrete texts and real-life experience.

Graumann (1989) has argued for an analysis of perspectivity in dialogue that sheds light on both perspective *setting* and perspective *taking* (cf. initiating and responding aspects). If we consider the global aspects of strongly asymmetrical interactions, we must then say that the subordinate party has very limited opportunities to set a perspective of his or her own. Sometimes, both parties (e.g. professional and layman) also have difficulties in *taking* the other's perspective.

It is obvious that many rights and responsibilities in social encounters cannot simply be derived from the roles of speaker versus addressee (versus other listeners). In fact, most obligative features seem to be tied to actor roles in specific activity types. In general, if we think of many institutional contexts, we find that the professional party is often charged with the responsibility of guaranteeing the outcome of the interaction (e.g. reaching a decision or getting certain information or advice across). This is often combined with a right – on the part of the professional – to decide which contributions are relevant and what is the 'correct' understanding of things talked about. As a result, the professional has a global responsibility for the whole encounter (forcing him to make some strong framing moves), while the client has only local responsibility of, e.g. answering the questions posed (Hobbs and Agar, 1985). This, no doubt, contributes to the fact that institutional discourse tends to exhibit asymmetries of several kinds (Agar, 1985).

Symmetrical and asymmetrical situations

There is a tendency within the social sciences to analyse social structures (and their micromanifestations in social encounters) either in terms of exchange relations or in terms of power relations. This seems to amount to isolating two types of interaction, one based on exchange and characterized by voluntariness, balance and symmetry, and one based on power and characterized by compulsion, imbalance and asymmetry. Following Baldwin (1978) and others, I would regard it as counterproductive to believe in two mutually exclusive families of situations. It is certainly true that situations vary in terms of asymmetry (or more accurately, different kinds of asymmetries), but all situations can be analysed both as exchange and power (or dominance). Direction, control and compliance, and initiative and response are always present in dialogue, and power relations are always to some extent intercursive.

The study of interactional patterns in different sorts of communicative activities might help us to construct a theory of social situations or, more accurately, dialogue participation structures. A very simple taxonomy might build upon the two dimensions of symmetry–asymmetry and co-operation–confrontation, and thus involve the following four ideal types:

1. The symmetrical-and-co-operative type(s).
2. The symmetrical-and-competitive type(s).
3. The asymmetrical-and-co-operative type(s).
4. The asymmetrical-and-competitive type(s).

The symmetrical-and-co-operative type(s) are collaborative and integrative in nature. Both parties are equally active, and the typical initiatives would be 'expanded responses' to the interlocutor's contributions, i.e. speakers both respond to what their partners have just said and introduce something new for them to respond to. Responses are invited rather than required. This seems to fit the ideal type of informal conversation between friends who are equally interested in maintaining their dialogue on topics with which they are equally familiar.

The symmetrical-and-competitive type(s) tend towards conflict and confrontation. Both parties are equally active, but they do not strive towards consensus. Instead, they pursue their own topics and argumentations (rather than jointly develop common understanding), and their interlocutor's initiatives are often ignored. The underlying logic, in extreme verbal disputes, may be one of emotional rather than cognitive coherence: you ignore the other's topic but respond to his or her accusation with a counter-accusation (Aronsson, 1987). Questions occur, especially challenging and meta-communicative ones (e.g. 'How can you say such a thing?').

The asymmetrical interactions are extremely common, particularly in situations where parties differ in status, competence and responsibilities. The asymmetrical-and-co-operative types, where most institutional interactions belong, are characterized by complementarity and divided responsibilities. One party takes the initiative and this is typically done by requesting (rather than just inviting) responses, i.e. by questions and directives, and the subordinate party tries to comply with the conditions, i.e. by answering questions and doing what he or she is told. In many cases, superior parties, e.g. professionals in institutional contexts, do provide some opportunities for subordinate parties to speak, but it is not uncommon that these opportunities remain unexploited. This then forces the superiors to return to more dominant actions, and the whole interaction reverts to asymmetries again.

In the asymmetrical-and-competitive type(s), the dominant party still takes the initiative (asks questions) but the subordinate party fails to comply, exhibiting instead some sort of passive resistance (reluctance to enter into the dialogue). According to our empirical evidence, such conditions seldom materialize in institutional contexts, at least not in routine tasks in a relatively consensus-oriented society like that of contemporary Sweden. Yet, some of our court trials (see Adelswärd, Aronsson and Linell, 1988) approach the characterization given here, be this due to genuine non-co-operation on the part of the defendants or to their relative unfamiliarity with the courtroom situation. Reluctance to engage in an interaction on the other's conditions is, however, not uncommon in many everyday situations. In fact, many quarrels seem to have their origin in such situations: one party is first reluctant to get involved and then, when sufficiently aroused, engages in a really confrontational interaction, which means that the parties have by then collectively moved over to a symmetrical-and-competitive-type situation. In terms of power relations, the asymmetrical-and-competitive-type situation is quite interesting. We have a dominant party, who tries to control the situation by taking strong measures, and a subordinate party, who uses the weapon of passive resistance, in itself a kind of power exercise. As a result, the dominant party is forced into a position of relative powerlessness, at least as far as the interactional outcome is concerned.

If we let the two dimensions cross-classify orthogonally and have different social situations located in the two-dimensional space thus created, we might end up with a diagram like Figure 2. Labels or concepts for 'social situation types' (such as those used in Figure 2) are assumed to be glosses or summaries derived on the basis of aggregates of microencounters. They belong to the (partially) shared representations of the social world which people have built up over a long time (see page 146).

Figure 2 is reminiscent of diagrams developed by Forgas (1979) on the basis of multidimensional scaling of people's assessments of different dyads on a battery of Osgood scales (Wish, Deutsch and Kaplan, 1976). Although so far Figure 2 has been based on intuitive judgements, it seems possible to secure an empirical underpinning for it; studies of actual interaction patterns would yield a basis for classifying social situations and their associated communicative activities. However, two dimensions would then almost certainly be insufficient. In fact, some inadequacies in Figure 2 are rather easily identifiable. For example, sales negotiations have been placed somewhere in the middle between friendly conversations between equals and verbal disputes, which is in some respects unsatisfactory.[8] Sales negotiations appear to involve a lot of mutual questioning which does not seem to be typical of either of the other two situation types. Like many other task-oriented encounters, sales negotiations seem to promote attempts at determining conditions for the contributions to come, i.e. demands for responses (questions). If we were to factor out this dimension (i.e. imposition versus non-imposition, or demanding (requesting) versus giving and inviting) and substitute as the third dimension straightness (versus obliqueness – where obliqueness, i.e. the opposite of straightness, involves avoiding giving straight responses to the interlocutor's preceding turns) we might get something like Table 3.

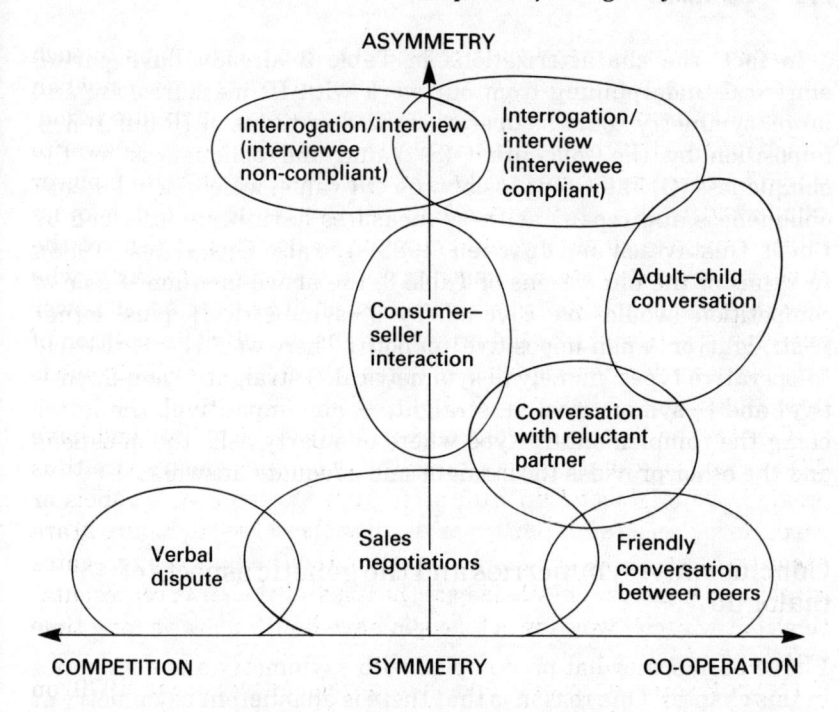

Figure 2 A simplified two-dimensional categorization of dyadic situations

Table 3 A three-dimensional analysis of some social situation types

	Symmetry[†]	Non-imposition	Straightness
Friendly conversation	+	+	+
Verbal dispute (quarrel)	+	+	−
Conversation with reluctant partner	−	+/−	+/−
Adult–child conversation	−	−	+(−)
Interview/interrogation:			
(a) with compliant interviewee	−*	−	+
(b) with non-compliant interviewee (passive resistance)	−	−	+/−
Sales negotiation	+	−	+/−
Consumer–expert/counsellor interview (active consumer)	+*/−	−	+

[†]This column concerns international (a)symmetry/dominance; especially in the cases asterisked (*), relationships may be reversed in terms of quantitative dominance (i.e. amount of talk).

In fact, the characterizations in Table 3 already have partial empirical underpinning from our work with IR measures. By and large, symmetry could be operationalized in terms of IR difference, imposition by the solicitation (S) value and obliqueness by the obliqueness (O) value (or possibly the OR value, which includes both obliqueness and repair) as these measures have been described by Linell, Gustavsson and Juvonen (1988) (see also Gustavsson, 1988). In terms of the dimensions of Table 3, the above-mentioned pole of competition would be covered by [+symmetrical] plus either [−straight] or [+non-impositive] (or both). There would be two clearly co-operative types, namely [+symmetrical, +straight, +non-impositive] and [−symmetrical, + straight, − non-impositive], the latter being the complementary type where one party asks the questions and the other provides the straight and adequate answers.

Conclusion: Asymmetries and the genetic aspects of dialogue

I have been somewhat preoccupied with asymmetry and dominance in this chapter. One reason is that there is an inherent asymmetry at the lowest level of dialogue, when − at each moment − one party keeps the floor and the other one stays on the outside (although he or she may contribute from his or her addressee position, through back-channelling and otherwise). Another reason is that many, in fact most, situations are also more or less asymmetrical at the level of activity and situation. In other words, asymmetries are present both locally (in individual utterances/turns) and globally (in sequences and whole dialogues/interactions/situations), i.e. at the two levels which have usually been regarded as fundamental to dialogue analysis.

In my view, the study of asymmetrical dialogues is a basic concern for dialogue theory. Yet some scholars, particularly some ethnomethodologists (see, e.g., Schegloff, 1987), have argued that it would be a healthy research strategy to stick to 'ordinary (or natural) conversation', at least for the foreseeable future. Presumably, 'ordinary conversation' is characterized by symmetry between the communicating parties and by the absence of particular constraints on topic choice and turn-taking (Atkinson and Heritage, 1984; Agar, 1985, p. 147). Luckmann (this volume, Chapter 2) reserves the term 'conversation' for this type of dialogue. Heritage summarizes some arguments for the primacy of this kind of dialogue as follows:

> Not only is 'ordinary conversation' the predominant medium of

interaction in the social world, it is also the primary form of interaction to which, with whatever simplifications, the child is first exposed and through which socialization proceeds. There is thus every reason to suppose that the basic forms of mundane talk constitute a kind of benchmark against which other more formal or 'institutional' types of interaction are recognized and experienced. (Heritage, 1987, p. 255)

In all fairness, it must be said that some Conversation Analysis scholars, including Heritage and Greatbatch (1989), have started working with institutional talk. However, while it must be conceded that there is a point in the argument quoted above, CA seems to fail to recognize that a good deal of informal, mundane conversation is characterized by asymmetries. In particular, the above socialization argument seems partly mistaken. In fact, infants and children are extremely dependent on their interlocutors in dialogue. As Rommetveit (1983) points out, children 'trade on adult truths', relying on their initiatives, meanings, knowledge and responsibility. Children start in a world of asymmetrical-and-co-operative situations, where adults dominate, even though they try to promote their young partners' development by expanding their responses (thus elaborating and upgrading the children's contributions) and perhaps by avoiding being overly impositive. Thus later, and only gradually, there will be a transition from other-regulation to more self-regulation and shared responsibility for contributing topics and perspectives; considerable time must elapse before the child can play the role of a fully capable and knowledgeable actor in friendly conversation on equal terms (the symmetrical-and-co-operative types), in the asymmetrical-and-competitive types (quarrels, arguing, 'sounding' etc.) and of course in the various institutional contexts that exist. Some of the latter, however, clearly involve the professional behaving as a parent providing protection and good advice.

Luckmann (this volume, Chapter 2) observes that the term 'conversation' (as used in the references given) would merely cover a range of particular, historical subspecies of 'dialogue'. There is no reason to assume that symmetrical talk-exchanges are necessarily universal. Still, even if there were something like 'ordinary conversations' in all human cultures, they would presumably constitute a minority of human dialogues. Asymmetries are probably more typical properties of dialogue than are symmetry and equality, at both local and global levels. Asymmetries inhere in both individual utterances (turns) and sequences. This makes them a natural focus in dialogue studies.

Notes

1. 'Dialogue' is taken to mean, roughly, any kind of talk exchange between two (or more) persons who are mutually co-present (Luckmann, this volume, Chapter 2). Hence, I do not include a condition of equality or symmetry in the definition.
2. All excerpts in this paper are rough, somewhat simplified, English translations of Swedish originals.
3. I take '(social) power' to be a relational concept pertaining to actor A's resources and means to influence actor B and his or her cognitions, emotions, actions and dispositions to act. This means that power is always present at a microlevel in communication. Several classical types of power prove to be essential: power in action (communication involves acting and attempts at having others act); power through knowledge (communication is largely a matter of having particular understandings and perspectives developed and endorsed); and systemic (organizational) power (actors are, to large but somewhat varying extents, the voices of cultures and traditions).
4. I disregard here the concept of 'dominance' as used in studies of non-verbal communication (as in human ethology and primatology). One might argue for the use of the term 'control' instead of 'dominance'. I shall, however, use 'control' in a narrower sense, referring to an actor's moves which attempt or serve to assess and reinterpret retroactively the other's contributions (involving acceptance or (re-)negotiation, ratification or disavowal etc.). (The corresponding future-oriented action would be directing and guiding.)
5. The excerpts given here are in fact much too short to allow for the calculation of reliable IR measures. For details of the coding scheme and analyses based upon it, I refer to Gustavsson (1988) and Linell, Gustavsson and Juvonen (1988).
6. Bakhtinian theory and down-to-earth coding schemes simply belong to quite different contexts of scientific use. Apparent differences are often due to different exigencies and divergent purposes. At a general level, it is true that every utterance has both a retrospective (response) aspect and a prospective (initiative) aspect. Still, when we want to measure and diagnose properties of individual authentic dialogues, it is nevertheless meaningful to say that some dialogue turns are pure responses and others pure initiatives – that is, if we restrict ourselves to the dialogue-internal (and local) ties between turns (Linell, Gustavsson and Juvonen, 1988).
7. The force of a local initiative is sometimes strong enough to break through firm and socially endorsed procedural rules. In particular, questions tend to get some kind of responses, whoever asks them. Thus, even in situations where the right to ask questions is preallocated to a superior party exclusively (e.g. to the judge or counsel in court, or to the interviewer in a news interview), if, occasionally, the other party (defendant, interviewee), asks a question, he will usually, at least after a repetition, get a response from the holder of the superordinate role (Adelswärd, Aronsson and Linell, 1988; Heritage and Greatbatch, 1989, p. 42).
8. For a study of sales negotiations, see Lampi (1986).

References

Adelswärd, V. (1988), *Styles of Success: On the collaborative presentation of self in job interviews*, Ph.D dissertation, University of Linköping: Linköping Studies in Arts and Science, 23.
Adelswärd, V., Aronsson, K., Jönsson, L. and Linell, P. (1987), 'The unequal distribution of interactional space: Dominance and control in courtroom interaction', *Text*, 7, 313–46.
Adelswärd, V., Aronsson, K. and Linell, P. (1988), 'Discourse of blame: Courtroom construction of social identity from the perspective of the defendant', *Semiotica*, 71, 261–84.
Agar, M. (1985), 'Institutional discourse', *Text*, 5, 147–68.
Aronsson, K. (1987), 'Verbal dispute and topic analysis. A methodological commentary on a drama case study', in F. van Zuuren, F. J. Wertz and B. Mook (eds), *Advances in Qualitative Psychology*, Swets & Zeitlinger.
Aronsson, K. and Rundström, B. (1988), 'Child discourse and parental control in pediatric consultations', *Text*, 8, 159–89.
Aronsson, K. and Sätterlund-Larsson, U. (1987), 'Politeness strategies and doctor–patient communication: On the social choreography of collaborative thinking', *Journal of Language and Social Psychology*, 6, 1–27.
Atkinson, M. and Heritage, J. (1984) (eds), *Structures of Social Action*, Cambridge: Cambridge University Press.
Bakhtin, M. M. (1986), *Speech Genres and Other Late Essays*, C. Emerson and M. Holquist (eds) trans. V. McGee, Austin: University of Texas Press.
Baldwin, D. (1978), 'Power and social exchange', *American Political Science Review*, 72, 1229–42.
Bales, R. F. (1950), *Interaction Process Analysis: A method for the study of small groups*, Reading, Mass.: Addison-Wesley.
Berger, P. and Luckmann, T. (1967), *The Social Construction of Reality*, Harmondsworth: Penguin.
Bruner, J. (1985), 'Vygotsky: A historical and conceptual perspective', in J. Wertsch (ed.), *Culture, Communication and Cognition: Vygotskian perspectives*, Cambridge: Cambridge University Press.
Cicourel, A. (1981), 'Notes on the integration of micro- and macro-levels of analysis', in K. Knorr-Cetina and A. Cicourel (eds), *Advances in Social Theory and Methodology: Toward an integration of micro- and macro-sociologies*, London: Routledge & Kegan Paul.
Danet, B. (1980), '"Baby" or "fetus"? Language and the construction of reality in a manslaughter trial', *Semiotica*, 32, 187–219.
Drew, P. (1985), 'Analyzing the use of language in courtroom interaction', in T. A. van Dijk (ed.), *Handbook of Discourse Analysis*, vol. 3: *Discourse and Dialogue*, New York: Academic Press.
Dunstan, R. (1980), 'Context for coercion: Analyzing properties of courtroom "questions"', *British Journal of Law and Society*, 6, 61–77.
Fillmore, C. J. (1985), 'Frames and the semantics of understanding', *Quaderni di Semantica*, 6(2), 222–54.
Forgas, J. (1979), *Social Episodes: The Study of Interaction Routines*, London: Academic Press.
Graumann, C. (1989), 'Perspective setting and taking in verbal interaction', in R. Dietrich and C. F. Graumann (eds), *Language Processing in Social Context*, Amsterdam: North Holland.

Gustavsson, L. (1988), *Language Taught and Language Used*, University of Linköping: Linköping Studies in Arts and Science, 18.
Heritage, J. (1984), *Garfinkel and Ethnomethodology*, Oxford: Polity Press.
Heritage, J. (1987), 'Ethnomethodology', in A. Giddens and J. Turner (eds), *Social Theory Today*, Cambridge: Polity Press.
Heritage, J. and Greatbatch, D. L. (1989), 'On the institutional character of institutional talk: The case of news interviews', forthc. in D. Boden and D. Zimmerman (eds), *Talk and Social Structure*, Oxford: Polity Press.
Heritage, J. and Sefi, S. (forthc.), '"Just a chat": health visitor–mother interaction in the home setting', forthc. in P. Drew and J. Heritage (eds), *Talk at Work*, Cambridge: Cambridge University Press.
Heritage, J. and Watson, R. (1980), 'Aspects of the properties of formulations in natural conversations: Some instances analysed', *Semiotica*, 30, 245–62.
Hobbs, J. R. and Agar, M. (1985), 'The coherence of incoherent discourse', *Journal of Language and Social Psychology*, 4, 213–32.
Hopper, R. (1983), 'Interpretation as coherence production', in R. T. Craig and K. Tracy (eds), *Conversational Coherence: Form, structure, and strategy*, Beverly Hills, Ca.: Sage.
Jönsson, L. (1988), *On Being Heard in Court Trials and Police Interrogations*, Ph.D dissertation, University of Linköping: Linköping Studies in Arts and Science, 25.
Lampi, M. (1986), *Linguistic Components of Strategy in Business Negotiations* (Studies B-85), Helsinki: School of Economics.
Linell, P. (1982), *The Written Language Bias in Linguistics*, Studies in Communication, SIC 2, Linköping: Department of Communication Studies.
Linell, P., Gustavsson, L. and Juvonen, P. (1988), 'Interactional dominance in dyadic communication: A presentation of initiative–response analysis', *Linguistics*, 26, 415–42.
Marková, I. (1982), *Paradigms, Thought and Language*, Chichester: Wiley.
Maturana, H. B. and Varela, F. (1980), *Autopoiesis and Cognition: The realization of the living*, Dordrecht: Reidel.
Maturana, H. B. and Varela, F. (1987), *The Tree of Knowledge. The Biological Roots of Human Understanding*, Boston, Mass.: New Science Library.
Mishler, E. G. (1984), *The Discourse of Medicine: Dialectics of medical interviews*, Norwood, N. J.: Ablex.
Pomerantz, A. (1984), 'Agreeing and disagreeing with assessments: Some features of preferred/dispreferred turn shapes', in J. M. Atkinson and J. Heritage (eds), *Structures of Social Action*, Cambridge: Cambridge University Press.
Reddy, M. (1979), 'The conduit metaphor – a case of frame conflict in our language about language', in A. Ortony (ed.), *Metaphor and Thought*, Cambridge: Cambridge University Press.
Rommetveit, R. (1974), *On Message Structure*, New York and Chichester: Wiley.
Rommetveit, R. (1983), 'In search of a truly interdisciplinary semantics: A sermon on hopes of salvation from hereditary sins', *Journal of Semantics*, 2, 1–28.
Rommetveit, R. (1987), 'Meaning, context, and control: Convergent trends and controversial issues in current social-scientific research on human cognition and communication', *Inquiry*, 30, 77–99.

Rommetveit, R. (1988a), 'On human beings, computers, and representational–computational versus hermeneutic–dialogical approaches to human cognition and communication', in H. Sinding-Larsen (ed.), *Artificial Intelligence and Language. Old Questions in a New Key*, Oslo: Tano.

Rommetveit, R. (1988b), 'On literacy and the myth of literal meaning', in R. Säljö (ed.), *The Written World*, Berlin: Springer, 13–40.

Rorty, R. (1979), *Philosophy and the Mirror of Nature*, Princeton, N. J.: Princeton University Press.

Schegloff, E. (1982), 'Discourse as an interactional achievement', in D. Tannen (ed.), *Analyzing Discourse: Text and Talk* (Georgetown University Round Table on Language and Linguistics, 1981), Washington, D.C.: Georgetown University Press.

Schegloff, E. (1987), 'Between Micro and Macro: Contexts and other connections, in J. Alexander, B. Giesen, R. Munch and N. Smelser (eds), *The Micro–Macro Link*, Los Angeles: University of California Press.

Schutz, A. (1967), *The Phenomenology of the Social World*, trans. G. Walsh and F. Lehnert (Northwestern University Studies in Phenomenology and Existential Philosophy), Evanston, Ill.: Northwestern University Press.

Searle, J. (1976), 'A classification of illocutionary acts', *Language in Society*, 5, 1–23.

Todorov, T. (1984), *Mikhail Bakhtin: The Dialogical Principle* trans. W. Godzich, Manchester: Manchester University Press.

Vološinov, V. N. (1973), *Marxism and the Philosophy of Language*, trans. L. Matejka and I. R. Titunik, New York: Seminar Press.

Wertsch, J. (1987), 'The role of voice in a sociocultural approach to mind', in W. Damon (ed.), *Child Development Today and Tomorrow*, San Francisco: Jossey-Bass.

Wish, M., Deutsch, M. and Kaplan, S. J. (1976), 'Perceived dimensions of interpersonal relations', *Journal of Personality and Social Psychology*, 33, 402–20.

Wrong, D. (1968), 'Some problems in defining social power', *The American Journal of Sociology*, 73, 673–81.

8 | Topic progression and intention

Klaus Foppa
Department of Psychology, University of Berne

Introduction

It is far from clear what is being referred to when speaking of 'the dynamics of dialogue'. The phrase is open to at least two different interpretations. The first rests on the assumption that any social encounter is of an interactive nature. Since 'interaction' refers to an ongoing process of mutual influence which in itself seems to be dynamic, it is quite natural to equate the interactive characteristics of dialogues with their dynamics. In this case, a demonstration that a social episode is interactive would of itself amount to proof that it is also dynamic. Of course, interaction itself is not as easily proven as one might assume. Usually it is overlooked that, for simple logical reasons, one has to consider at least three behavioural 'steps' in order to make inferences about the interactive nature of a sequence of social events. These steps are: a first action by a person A (a1), the temporally following action of person B (b1), and the temporally subsequent action of person A (a2) (Foppa, 1978; Heritage, 1984; Käsermann, 1980 (1978); Marková, 1987, this volume, Chapter 6; Mead, 1934). Taking into account only two behavioural acts, say a1 and b1 (in this temporal order), could at best show some influence of a1

I would like to thank several colleagues for their very valuable and helpful comments, especially Marie-Louise Käsermann, Ivana Marková, and Theres Mühlemann. Without Ivana Marková's assistance and the advice of Colin Wright of the University of Exeter concerning matters of English language, the paper would not have got its present form. However, none of them should be too disappointed if the result is not up to their expectations.

on b1 (or of person A on person B) but it could show no influence whatsoever of person B on person A.

A second interpretation of the phrase 'the dynamics of dialogue' is not primarily concerned with interactivity. Consider the following example. One of the participants in a dialogue has a single goal in mind, that of ensuring that the future course of action will depend on his or her own decision alone. No matter what plans the partner may have, this participant will seek to thwart them and secure his or her own intentions instead. Note that in this case the dynamic nature of the dialogue cannot be attributed to its interactive aspects in general. Instead, it rests on the firm and determined intentions of *one* of the interactants. He or she is held responsible for the *dynamic impression* of the whole process. And the other participant of these verbal exchanges *experiences* their dynamic nature either because he or she simply is aware of the partner's intentions or because he or she attributes certain intentions to the partner, depending on his or her expectations.

However, this does not mean that the communicators' intentions have to be very explicit or even very specific. It suffices that at least one of the communicators tries hard to make him- or herself understood or to understand what has been said. As soon as one of them has difficulties in getting a message through, he or she may, for example, start to speak louder and in a more articulated manner rephrase his or her utterances again and again, correct misunderstandings etc., depending on the specific characteristics of the situation (Käsermann, 1980 (1978); Käsermann and Foppa, 1981; Clark and Schaefer, 1989). Frequently, these types of behaviour do not seem to be based on very specific goals. Nevertheless, they are usually 'explained' in terms of 'communicative intentions': people behave in the way they do *because* of their (assumed) *intentions* to inform another person, to understand what others say, etc.

Such 'explanations' may look satisfying to the layperson, but psychologists have difficulties in accepting them as being scientific. not so much because they do not like the idea that 'intentionality' (see Luckmann, this volume, Chapter 2) may be an essential and general feature of human nature. The crucial problem has to do with the fact that, despite a growing interest in the concept of 'intention' as such (see action theories, for example Cranach *et al.*, 1981; or motivation theories, for example Halisch and Kuhl, 1987), there are no satisfactory empirical methods, either for the identification of different intentional states, or for the scientific 'proof' of intentions in other persons. This seems to be due to a certain vagueness in the concept of intention, which is less unequivocal than it may seem at first sight.

Although one can easily understand that statements like: 'I didn't want to hurt you!', 'I'll give it to you tomorrow' or 'I am determined to quit my job' have as reference certain *intentional states*, the reference to the speakers' intentions is, in fact, *twofold*:

1. The speaker may want to give you certain information, i.e. make a specific statement (in terms of speech act theory, perform a *propositional act* – see, e.g., Searle, 1969); or
2. He or she may make the utterance *in order* to convince you, to make a promise, etc., thereby performing an *illocutionary act* (*ibid.*).

The intention to convey a certain message (and not another one), i.e. the intention in the propositional sense or '*what*' *intention*, is quite different from the intention to say something in order to get at a certain 'strategic' goal, i.e. the intention in the illocutionary sense or '*what for*' *intention*. The difference becomes clear as soon as one tries to find out what a person intended to say. One's immediate reaction might simply be to ask him or her: 'What did you want to say when you said X?'. But very probably one would get an answer like the following: 'I wanted to say X' or a paraphrase of X. Note that one is forced into circularities of language as soon as one starts this kind of inquiry. Since one does not have any more valid information about the person's 'what' intention with respect to the utterance 'I wanted to say X' than with respect to the preceding utterance 'X', one is led to ask further questions, such as: 'What did you want to say when you said "I wanted to say X"?', and so on. Certainly it may sometimes be possible to answer the question by gestures, but usually there is no other way of informing another person about one's 'what' intentions than by verbalizing them (James, 1890). It is only by more *indirect ways* that one can get at the core of what a person has intended to say. Imagine a series of *self- or other-repairs*: besides the question of their possible function in conversation (Schegloff, 1979), one may treat them as attempts at the verbalization of a certain message, i.e. at the realization of a specific 'what' intention. This intention may be inferred from the different attempts either by focusing on their invariant parts or by taking together what has been said in the individual repairs (Foppa, 1984). Take the following two examples.

I
M: I said I'd never *do* that, I'm *say*ing though, I'm saying I've had all kinds o' opportunities 'n I've never *done* it, that's what I was *say*ing.

(Crow, 1983, p. 146)

The 'core' of this message, which can be taken as equivalent to the speaker's 'what' intention, can be formulated in the following way:
I said (I'm saying)/
I'd never do that (I've never done it)
(though) (I've had all kinds o' opportunities).

The second example is different from the first.

II
A: This place reminds me of that restaurant, remember, Our House?
W: What? This reminds you of our house?
A: No! The restaurant Our House.
W: Our house?
A: No, that restaurant where we ate pie, over by Baskin Robbins, with a lot of older people.
W: Oh.

(Beach, 1983, p. 202)

Here, the misunderstanding by W forces A to make more and more explicit what he or she meant by, or wanted to say with, 'that restaurant, remember, Our House'.

It is not these 'what' intentions and the possibilities of their identification that I shall deal with in this chapter. Although they are pertinent to those aspects of *dialogical dynamism* which rest on the co-operative efforts of the participants (Foppa, 1984, 1987a; Foppa and Käsermann, 1981; Käsermann, 1980 (1978)), I shall focus here on the 'what for' intentions and their role in the dynamics of dialogue. In justification of this it is sufficient to point to the fact that one can easily overlook the *fundamental* conceptual and methodological *differences* between the two types of intentions – Cranach (1986) and Foppa (1987b) being a good example of a controversy caused by a lack of differentiation between them.

Given one's interest in the 'what for' intention of another person, one might simply *ask* him or her: '*Why* did you say this?'. Note that this would not lead into language circularities as neither repeating nor paraphrasing an utterance would constitute an appropriate answer to the 'why' question. Of course, if a speaker is aware of his or her reasons and willing to talk about them it is feasible to ask directly. But one can never be quite sure whether this is the case or not and it is impossible to rely on persons' statements about their ability and readiness to disclose their goals. As with 'what' intentions – but for different reasons – one has to use more *indirect* methods.

One may speculate about the possible influences of certain 'what for' or *strategical* or *interactive* intentions on the course of a dialogue. Imagine a person who wants to find out whether his or her partner is really interested in getting a specific job. Probably, he or she will try to bring up the topic of interest again and again (thus displaying its 'dynamic force'). As a consequence, such a dialogue would have to show a different pattern of topic progression from that in a dialogue in which none of the participants is aiming at specific goals, e.g. party conversations. I will come back to this point after having dealt with some aspects of topic progression in general.

Some general aspects of topic progression

Topic progression seems to be one of the *constitutive features* of dialogues. Verbal exchanges which show no kind of topic development can hardly be perceived as 'natural' conversations. Imagine two people conversing together. Suppose that they talk in a regular fashion, i.e. they take turns according to the rules, and that their utterances are more or less coherent, i.e. the utterances are somehow related to one another. Perhaps, however, what the speakers contribute to the conversation are only repetitions of their respective former utterances. Such a 'conversation' could read as follows:

III
 A: I shall go to Zurich.
 B: And I'll go to Geneva.
 A: I shall go to Zurich.
 B: And I'll go to Geneva.
 A: I shall go to Zurich.
etc.

It is only under very specific conditions that a dialogue like this could take place. And it would be absolutely unnatural unless the lack of topic development were compensated for by certain *co-verbal* aspects like intonation, stress and loudness. One could imagine two boys quarrelling with each other, and repeating again and again their statements, except that, for example, they spoke more and more loudly as they went on. Interestingly, even in this case we get the impression of two persons whose actions are determined by certain interactive, strategic or 'what for' intentions. The fact that the interlocutors speak louder and louder would make us believe that they are, for example, trying to *dominate* each other. This inference seems to be straightforward and one may be misled into assuming that it is always these co-verbal (and non-verbal) parameters which are responsible for our inferences about the communicators' intentions. Nevertheless, some caution seems to be warranted. One must not overlook the fact that the meaning of these co-verbal signals, despite their persuasiveness, has still to be proved.

Fortunately, conversations are usually not as monotonous as our imaginary example. And, besides, the interlocutors themselves do not rely exclusively on non- or co-verbal means to get at their interactive or strategic goals. The two communicators in example III would probably not only speak louder and louder but try to accomplish their respective goals *verbally*. If they were interested in convincing each other that their own choice of destination were the preferable one, the conversation might develop as follows:

IV
A: I shall go to Zurich.
B: And I'll go to Geneva.
A: But Zurich is more interesting.
B: That may be true but Lac Leman is much more beautiful than the Zürichsee.
A: OK. But what are you going to do when it is raining?
etc.

Irrespective of the questionable naturalness of this bit of conversation, there is no doubt that 'what for' intentions do manifest themselves in real dialogues in this way. This is not at all astonishing since there are not many possibilities for their manifestation. Thus a person who is really concerned to convince another of something can only try out a limited set of possible lines of attack: for example, he or she can reject the counter-arguments of the interlocutor, or bring up new aspects, or refer to new material, etc. This has two possible consequences. First, it leads to a certain dialogue *structure*, i.e. both participants sticking to a certain topic as long as they believe they have been unsuccessful in attaining their respective goals, and as long as they continue their conversation and do not (explicitly) change its topic. Second, since the topic must be changed or at least new aspects of it must be introduced if it is referred to unduly, a certain 'movement' or *development* is inevitably contributed to it.

But the simple fact of *topic progression* must not always be taken as evidence that the interlocutors have specific intentions in mind. Topic development may occur without any very concrete intentions. Think again of party conversations. People speak to each other, obviously without any fixed goal. They simply try to avoid long pauses and risky topics. It would be misleading to infer any specific strategic goals from the fact that their talk, nevertheless, does 'proceed'.

In order to understand the more complex mechanisms of topic developments as consequences of specific strategic intentions, it seems necessary to establish something like a 'base-level' of conversational progression. In other words, one should learn more about topic change without specific intentions before dealing more extensively with the other forms. In the following section, therefore, I will deal with the mechanisms of *topic management in small talk*. Only then will I proceed to the more interesting questions of the role of intentions and how they manifest themselves in the course of communicative interaction.

Speaking without specific intentions and the local management of topic development

Informal conversations such as party talk have one feature in common: the participants start talking about something, and after a short while they talk about something completely different. Mostly, there are smooth changes of topic aspects which are barely detectable but which nevertheless eventually lead to something 'new'. However, one does not get the impression that speakers *plan* to proceed in a particular way, or know in advance what they are going to say, or for what reason. As mentioned above, the bridging of pauses and the avoidance of conflict frequently seem to be the only interest of the interlocutors. (For reasons of simplicity I leave aside the personal interests that participants may have in each other.) The *topic changes* seem to come about in an unplanned manner, by themselves, as it were.

There are different ways in which this may happen. In any turn of a certain minimal length the speaker him- or herself produces topic progression with respect to his or her own former utterances. Topic progression in this sense refers to a turn-internal process. It reflects a sort of dynamic aspect of dialogue which may be called *monologic*, insofar as it rests primarily on the speaker him- or herself. It is true that this is not monologic in the full sense of the word since the mere presence of a partner influences the way in which the single utterances follow each other. But it points to the fact that it is predominantly the speaker him- or herself who decides the course of the development (but see Bergman's concept of 'local sensitivity', this volume, Chapter 9). This decision process is of some interest. Frequently the speakers are neither totally aware of it (in the sense of anticipating the wording of their later utterance) nor do they proceed purely by chance. They seem to be guided by rather vague 'what' intentions which are defined *ex negativo*, so to say. This means that the speakers in fact do not know in advance what they are going to say but immediately notice when they have 'lost' their topic or have not really said what they – paradoxically – 'wanted' to say.

Of course, I am not suggesting that there are no situations in which the speakers know very well what they are going to say *before* they start speaking. Prepared speeches are a good example. In this case speakers document their preparedness by using notes or scripts to which they refer whenever they are not quite sure how to continue. Nevertheless, whenever they produce an utterance of their talk *in situ*, it will show structural similarities to the monologic phases in dialogues, and the process of construction seems to be similar in both cases. However, before I go on to demonstrate some of the characteristics of this process I must deal with certain technical problems.

One of the difficulties in analysing spoken language arises from the fact that one does not usually speak in complete sentences. Certainly, there are segments which are marked, e.g. by pauses, or by their intonation contour or by certain structural features which remind one of something like sentences. But since there is no generally agreed method for segmentation, one satisfies oneself with partitioning the individual contributions into turns. However, this way of partitioning conversations is obviously too rough to be sensitive to the questions of psychological interest, and it is not well suited to the analysis of monologic phases.

The method of segmenting transcripts proposed by Moesch (1987) in my view offers a solution to this problem. It is simple, easy to apply and sufficiently objective and reliable. The single segments, which are called analytic units (AUs), seem to reflect psychologically relevant aspects of the processes of production and reception, and of the interlocutors' communicative interaction (Mühlemann and Foppa, 1989). The units are based on the verbs (the grammatical predicates), i.e. it is always the verb which is taken as the *core* of any AU. In V the result of this procedure is demonstrated. (AUs are marked by / at their beginning and end.)

V
A: /*Did* you *remember*/
   /that broccoli *is* the second most nutritious vegetable?/
W: /To what?/ (Ellipsis)

A: /What?/
W: /To what?/
A: /I *don't understand*./
W: /Well, if broccoli *is* the second most nutritious
    vegetable/
    /what's *the first?*/
A: Oh, tha : : :t's/
    /what you *mean*!/
    /I *didn't understand*/
    /what you *were getting at*./
    /Collard greens *are* more nutritious than broccoli./

(Beach, 1983, pp. 202f.)

As one can easily see, the analytic units consist of the verb and those parts of the respective utterance which are immediately related to it. Of course there are exceptions, ellipses, for example. Moesch has proposed a set of rules which allows for the handling of a great variety of very specific cases such as ellipses and other verbless utterances. For present purposes, however, it suffices to consider the most important aspects of this 'pragmatic procedure'.

Let us come back to the problems of turn-internal and monological topic progression. Wunderlich (1976) reports the beginning of a talk delivered by the German linguist John Gumperz who at that time had lived in the United States for many years. One would presume him to have become a fluent English speaker by now and he had published regularly in English. However, the talk began in the following way:

VI
/ahh. what. I thought/
/I would talk to you about today./
/is ah. ah I would give you that I would give you a
    preliminary report of some of the field work/
/that I have been doing in England for the last ah last
    four or five months.../
/and this is work/
/that comes out of ah my interest originally came out of
    my interest in sociolinguistics ah specifically
    out of my interest in code switching.../
/ah I've been interested for quite some time in ah in
    the use of two or three languages in conversation
    as a means of communication/
etc. (Wunderlich, 1976, p. 345)

Reading the AUs one after the other, one gets the impression that each of them is in some way or another a *continuation* or *expansion* of something said in one of the *immediately antecedent* AUs. For example, the last AU:

/ah I've been interested for quite some time in ah in the use of two or three languages in conversation as a means of communication/

gives an *explanation* of the kind of code switching the speaker has referred to in the preceding AU. The AU:

/that comes out of ah my interest originally came out of my interest in sociolinguistics ah specifically out of my interest in code switching.../

can be understood as an additional comment on the fieldwork he has spoken about in:

/is ah.ah I would give you that I would give you a preliminary report of some of the field work/.

This leads to a gradual increase in specification in the speaker's talk about his research interests, as Wunderlich (1976, p. 348) points out:

my interest
my interest in sociolinguistics
my interest in code switching
I've been interested in the use of two or three languages in
      conversation as a means of communication
what I have been interested in in working with code switching (is)
      the semantic content of code switching
what I've been interested in are the conditions.

Note, that it is also a very simple and effective means of bringing about topic progression. Certainly, it presupposes at least something like a very general lead on the speaker's side, but in its details it is accomplished by taking up 'local' aspects and 'following' their direction.

Turn-internal topic management in a dialogical situation seems to function in a very similar way. In example VII I have emphasized those parts to which each AU immediately refers, and have put them in front of their respective AUs. The numbers in parentheses refer to the turn numbers in Craig and Tracy (1983):

VII

(207) *K*: /When I was home, two years ago/
       (*when I was home*) / they flooded really bad. A-at Christmas time. No at spring break/
       (*they flooded really bad*) /And one of the roads we=

(208) *B*:   ((laugh))

(209) *K*:   =had to go – through/
       (*one of the roads we had to go through*) / to get back up to Wisconsin/
       (*one of the roads*) /was: oh: maybe twenty feet above the riv- above the river in Iowa./
       (*above the river*) /it wasn't the main river, but a small river./
       (*a small river*) /and it was flooded over with at least a foot of water/
       (*it was flooded with at least a foot of water*)/ and this was after it had gone down a lot./
       (*195 (!) it's four large cities*) /There's just so – but there's so much to *do* in these towns/

etc.

                                                (Craig and Tracy, 1983, p. 313)

There is only one deviation from the linguist's pattern in topic development (example VI), namely the last AU in which the speaker refers to a topic previously spoken about in turn number 195. As I will maintain later on, such deviations from the simple pattern of *local continuation* always point to a different mechanism of topic progression which rests on specific 'what' or 'what for' intentions of the respective speaker.

Topic changes do not come about by turn-internal processes alone. alone. Speakers not only expand what they themselves have said before but usually refer to the interlocutor's utterances as well. If the avoidance of conflicts is the primary goal of a communicator only a rather restricted set of possible continuations can be considered. To something one has already said one can only make an addition, make a comment or give an explanation; otherwise one can only ask questions or confirm one's partner's statements. Any other continuation would either amount to a change of topic, or to an infringement of this *principle of neutral local coherence*. This holds true for contradictions, rejections or corrections. But even justificatory remarks are problematic because they may be interpreted as defensive.

Example VIII shows a rather typical turn-internal and dialogical topic development in a conversation in which the interlocutors seem to have no specific goals in mind. The numbers which directly precede the AUs in K's turn mark their reverse temporal position: the last AU has the number (1), the last but one the number (2), and so on. K's AUs are added in the analysis of B's turn insofar as B's AUs relate to them. This makes it easier to show that any particular utterance usually refers to one of the interlocutor's last AUs. Again, the emphasized expressions in parentheses indicate the parts of the speaker's own former utterances to which he or she is referring.

VIII
(213) *K*: ...
(6) / and it starts over at one,/
(*and it starts over at one*) (5)/ but – they're still, like the ones that – run parallel, through the towns,/
(*the ones that run parallel through the towns*)
(4)/ are – seventeen and seventeen, twenty-three and twenty-three/
(*3rd AU of (213)*: *I don't get lost down there*) (3) / an' it's – just – you can't get lost/
(*you can't get lost*) (2) / Until you go into Davenport./
(*until you go into Davenport*) (1) / And ((laughing)) then you can get lost./
(214) *B*: ((laugh...) (pause))
(2) (*until you go into Davenport*) / I wasn't – driving when we went there/
(1) (*then you can get lost*) / so I didn't think about getting lost, you know,/
(*I wasn't driving*) / somebody else dealt with ((laughing)) those things./
etc.

(Craig and Tracy, 1983, pp. 313f.)

Topic progression seems to be brought about in the dialogical situation in the same manner as in the monological or in the turn-internal case, that is *locally*. This means at least that people who do not have very specific 'what for' intentions or strategic goals seem to construct their conversational contributions in a rather *ad hoc* manner. Reading the references and the AUs together gives one the impression of an almost perfect fit between the string of words in square brackets and the following AU. This might reflect nothing more than the principle according to which the references are selected. But it could also be a manifestation of the speaker's tendency for 'piecemeal construction of ideas while speaking' (i.e. Kleist's (1886–90) 'allmähliche Verfertigung der Gedanken beim Reden'). By simply taking one aspect of a former utterance as the starting point for what follows, one has already automatically started to exhaust the possible meanings of a given topic, and initiated topic progression. The direction this progression takes seems to depend – at least in small talk – on the elements of that AU. The exact route of continuation is therefore scarcely predictable. It depends, additionally, on the prevailing specific conditions which comprise the speakers' linguistic competence, their general knowledge, their actual emotional state, their social relationship (e.g. its asymmetry – Linell, this volume, Chapter 7), their shared knowledge (Rommetveit, 1968) and their perspective on reality (Graumann, 1989; this volume, Chapter 5).

The most important difference between the monological and turn-internal mechanisms of topic progression on the one hand and the dialogical ones on the other seems to lie in the probability of new topic elements being introduced. As soon as *two* people are responsible for the management of topic progression, greater variability in the aspects which are expanded from AU to AU can be expected. As a consequence, the topic span of dialogues should – *ceteris paribus* – be much broader than that of (real) monologues.

The effectiveness of *local topic management* in small talk is beyond question, and its functioning is not at all surprising. Since the interlocutors are concerned to avoid conflicts, the listener looks for the chance of a turn only when the speaker mentions something on which he or she feels able to comment unobtrusively. This gives rise to the 'last come, first served' principle, i.e. to the neutral local coherence principle mentioned above.

However, even in small talk there are additional mechanisms to be considered. There are various effective means of directing the course of the conversation, and of thereby influencing the development of topics. Questions, which are one example, do not necessarily reflect any real interest on the part of the questioner; they can be simply a communicative routine to maintain an ongoing conversation. Nevertheless, even the location of questions seems to follow (at least in 'intention-free' communication) the same principle: questions are addressed at those aspects of the partner's preceding utterance which it seems harmless to address. A second example is the various means of securing mutual understanding, such as paraphrasing an interlocutor's utterance by saying: 'Am I correct in understanding your utterance as X?', where X is a paraphrase. Inevitably, this leads to an elaboration of meanings and to an expansion of topic aspects, thereby bringing about topic development.

In concluding these considerations about certain mechanisms of topic progression in general, I wish to stress again the possibility of topic changes occurring without any specific intentions on the part of the interlocutors. In the following section I will try to show in a more detailed way how deviations from this principle of *neutral local coherence* and *local topic management* can be taken as indications of more or less specific intentional states of the communicators.

Topic progression as the result of 'intentional' speaking

While in 'intention-free' or aimless conversations the participants seem to follow the flow of utterances in much the same way as an unsteered boat follows the course of a river, things are quite different as soon as either or both of them has a certain goal 'in mind'. This may concern the *content of* as well as the *reason for* the verbal exchange in question. It is especially this latter aspect which I will deal with in this section.

I shall assume that any violation of the principle of neutral local coherence is prima facie reason for supposing that the violator has a certain *strategic intention*. This conjecture is based on rather simple logic: neutral local coherence as sketched above, i.e. simply continuing, expanding or explaining the last parts of preceding utterances, cannot be maintained throughout a dialogue or any conversation once the speaker wants to get to a certain point. It is highly improbable that, for example, negotiations of any kind could proceed in the 'last come, first served' manner. Instead, one will have to expect at least some disagreement, some corrections, some counter-arguments, etc.

Naturally, violations of the principle of neutral local coherence can only indicate the strategic intention as such, without saying anything about the *specific goals* which the speaker is aiming at. But at least some of the specific interactive intentions are easy to identify. Take the following example (IX), which represents the questioning of a defendant (D) by his defence lawyer (DL). (In contrast to the original transcript, the reproduced one is partitioned into AUs.)

IX
The defendant is accused of having rented video boxes and other goods and then sold them to get money for paying back a debt

DL: /Did you know/
/or had you rented any such boxes before?/
D: /No, no no that.../
DL: /So it was this person, your creditor,/
/who who told you/
/how you should go about doing it and...?/
D: /Yes, he said so, you know,/
/now you've got your chance and so.../
/He knew it,/
/so you have just to step in/
/and rent this, or something like that./
DL: /But did you realize/
/that by writing your name on those um.../
D: /Oh yes, I realized/
/that I would end up here in court, you know,/
/and have to get things straight, you know, but anyway.../
DL: /But you mean/
/that um the alternative was/
/to be struck half dead/
/if you did...?/
D: /Well, half, wholly maybe/
DL: /and you had no other possibilities/
/to get your money?/
D: /I called my mum/
/and tried to borrow money,/
/but there was no way there either./

(Trial, No. 41: 30–1; Linell, this volume, Chapter 7)

The *deviations* from the principle of neutral local coherence in this example are obvious. It is also obvious that the defence lawyer at least, is *aiming at something*. As Linell notes: 'In this case we see a defence lawyer using his privileged position to invoke a perspective on events talked about, and this was in the interest of his client and interactant' (*ibid.*, p. 163). I think one can easily agree with this interpretation. But how do we know that we are right? Is it simply our understanding of the English language which justifies our attribution of this specific goal to the defence lawyer? Or is it our general knowledge of the behaviour of defence lawyers which entitles us to make the attribution?

Closer inspection of the dialogue (IX) reveals some interesting details. It is not only that the defence lawyer asks one question after another, but the way these questions follow the defendant's answers, and the way the individual topics are introduced are significant. The defence lawyer does not, in a small talk fashion, take up some aspect of what the defendant has said, but seems to follow a certain line of argumentation almost without dwelling on the details of the defendant's answers. Take for example the first few lines of the interrogation:

DL: /Did you know/
/or had you rented such boxes before?/
D: No, no no that..../
DL: So it was this person, your creditor,/
/who who told you/
/how you should go about doing it and...?/

Taking up the defendant's answer to his first question, the defence lawyer gives a very specific interpretation to it. He does not simply continue what the defendant has said, but suggests instead, as Linell notes, a particular perspective on certain events. Note that it is not yet clear what the defence lawyer is aiming at. So far we can only say that he does not obey the principle of neutral local coherence.

Let us look at the defence lawyer's questions put in sequence:

Did you know or had you rented any such boxes before?
So it was this person, your creditor, who who told you how
    you should go about doing it and...?
But did you realize that by writing your name on those
    you um...
    D: *Oh yes, I realized that I would end up*
    here in court, you know, and have to get
    things straight, you know, but anyway...
But you mean that um the alternative was to be struck
    half dead if you did...?
and you had no other possibilities to get your money?

Without knowing the defendant's answers (with one single exception which is necessary for an adequate understanding of the ongoing exchange), the sequence of the defence lawyer's questions shows clearly the *gist* of his intervention. At the same time it gives an idea of his *strategic intentions*, which could be summarized as follows:

> Your creditor told you how to proceed, and although you were aware of the dangers of your doing so you saw no other possibilities of getting the necessary money.

That is probably what the defence lawyer wanted to say. Taking the context into account, one can suppose that he wanted to say it for the simple reason of convincing the court that the defendant was *not* to blame for the crime in question. Note that one does not need to do much interpretative work to get at this point, and that one stays more or less at the surface of the utterances. One cannot infer any underlying intentions by this line of reasoning. If, for example, the defence lawyer wasn't really seeking to convince the court of the defendant's relative innocence but was behaving in every way as if he were, this fact could not be discovered. Speakers' 'hidden motives' remain in the dark and there is no torch at hand to illuminate the darkness.

Courtroom dialogues are probably not the best examples for a discussion of the problems which arise in the context of analyses of strategical intentions. Since the respective roles of the interlocutors are clear from the very beginning, their intentions are too: a defence lawyer has, almost 'by definition', to defend his or her client, and this is at least one of the underlying intentions of his or her actions. Let me therefore refer to a different type of example (X). It is taken from the transcript of a psychotherapeutic session with a girl who lived with her divorced father.

X

Therapist: /Well, I'm aware/
/that you really feel sometimes/
/that you are kind of neglected/
Julie: /Yeah, a lot/
Therapist: /You don't live with your mom and your dad,/
/so you kind of miss out on having two parents./
/You do have one parent/
/who loves you very much,/
/but you don't really get to see him./
Julie: /My father . . . every night practically, he goes to the city/
/because my grandma's home./
/She's visiting from Florida./

                /Gosh, last night he said/
                /he would be home early./
                /You know he likes to go out to dinner./
                /He didn't get home until real late./
                /I didn't get to see him/
                /before I went to sleep./
Therapist: /And then what happens is/
                /when you do get his attention/
                /it is always a kind of negative attention./
                /He's angry at you or .../
Julie: /... if he's home,/
                /he's watching TV or he's .../
Therapist: /... upset with you?/
Julie: /Right./
                /Or if he's out/
                /he's out all night/
                /and he never comes home./
Therapist: /So that is very difficult for you./

(Morawetz and Walker, 1984, p. 266)

Take the first of Julie's somewhat longer turns (/My father... every night practically, he goes to the city/ etc.), and the therapist's reply (/And then what happens is/ etc.). Of course, this somehow *continues* Julie's complaints about her father. But it does not need very close inspection to note that it is *not the neutral continuation* of 'intention-free' conversations. Violation of the neutral local coherence principle always points to some specific strategic intention of the violator. However, it is only the *specific relationship* between the violator's utterance and the statement of the interlocutor to which it refers, or the kind of topic progression, respectively, which renders possible inferences about the kind of strategic intention the violator has. It is for this reason that one may take the following set of AUs as a kind of interpretative summary or generalization of what Julie has said (and what the therapist already knows about the whole situation).

/And then what happens is/
/when you do get his attention/
/it is always a kind of negative attention./
/He's angry at you or .../
...
/... upset with you?/
...
/So that is very difficult for you./

Furthermore, it is because of our general knowledge of therapeutic settings that we can assume that the therapist is acting in pursuit of certain therapeutic goals, for example to explain the meaning of a given situation.

Different as the two examples (IX) and (X) may be, they have one important characteristic in common. In both dialogues interactive intentions may be seen as more or less *conscious goals* of action on which the actors would probably be able to comment *in advance*. Since these strategic or interactive intentions are identified on the basis of violations of or deviations from the principle of neutral local coherence, one might be misled into assuming that any deviation from this principle points to some sort of conscious strategic intention and that the dynamics of dialogue which seems to be so closely related to the interlocutors' 'what for' intentions is therefore simply a matter of conscious control. This is certainly not the case.

Let us consider another interesting example (XI) of a conversation which shows deviations from neutral local coherence. These deviations are hardly to be attributed to conscious strategic intentions.

XI
H: /Look/
/I just wish/
/you would tell me/
/what I've done wrong – /
/I mean/
/you're so damned angry!/
S: /Well, I'm not even sure/
/I remember exactly/
/what it was;/
/it was everything;/
/you just really pissed me off,/
/that's all – /
/Anyway, I don't want/
/to keep going through it . . ./
/I'm – ((Interruption))/
H: /You're the one/
/that keeps – /((Interruption))
S: I'm saying things/
/I don't even mean./
/Look,/
/ask me tomorrow – /
/I'm sorry,/
/I just lost it there for a while . . ./
H: /Ok./

(Farrell, 1983, p. 272)

According to H's first question, S seems to be rather angry. /You just really pissed me off,/ is a description of his anger which certainly has no place in 'intention-free' dialogues, and at the same time is not due to a considerate, conscious and elaborated strategic intention of the speaker. Instead, it is probably no more than the expression of an *emotional state*.

Such *emotional responses* seem to be at least as important for the development of conversations as the more 'intellectual' strategic intentions. They are of central importance for the dynamic nature of dialogues. Nevertheless, we do not know much about the specific conditions under which they occur, and we have no very precise idea about the way they function. Suffice it to say that there are deviations from the principle of neutral local coherence which are not to be understood as consequences of the interlocutors' strategic intentions.

While the interlocutors are, at least to a certain degree, *aware* of their emotional states, even if they do not want to report on them, there are other examples of deviations from neutral local coherence which are neither the result of strategic intentions nor the expression of a specific emotional state. Käsermann has recently (Käsermann and Altorfer, 1989a, 1989b) examined phenomena of this kind. Interlocutors may communicate with each other in a *non-co-operative* way, using very subtle means to hinder their partner(s) from participating in the conversation in an adequate way. Käsermann therefore speaks of the obstruction and impediment which may be exerted in conversations. It is to be doubted whether people usually hinder their partners intentionally (in the full sense of the word) and consciously. Nevertheless, the impediments seem to induce physiological stress (Käsermann and Altorfer, 1989a), which means that they in fact function as if the speaker had intended to produce these effects. It may therefore be appropriate to speak of the *functional effectiveness* of these (unintentional) communicative strategies. Needless to say, like the above-mentioned emotional responses, these communicative strategies add substantially to the dynamics of the conversation (see Käsermann and Altorfer, 1989b).

Before I come to my concluding remarks there is one very general rider which I wish to add. At best one may find these speculations less than fully convincing. 'But,' somebody may ask, 'where is the necessary experimental evidence? Do you have any statistically significant results?' This critic may continue. 'Your examples are very interesting but they are no more than illustrative examples. Aren't there any other, somewhat "harder", data?'. I would have to confess that not only can I not offer any such empirical results, but I am also very sceptical about the very possibility of strictly experimental investigations in this domain. What is more, I see no way of defining populations from which (representative) samples could be drawn, such that one could make statistical inferences about the probabilities of Null hypotheses (Foppa, 1987c). Even if I am not right about this, I do not see how any experiments could be designed except on the basis of some observations and tentative speculations. I believe that my conjectures about the function of intentions and the possibilities of their identification should be taken seriously, at least as suggestions for further empirical research.

Conclusion

In this chapter I have tried to demonstrate several things. First, I have speculated about the close relationship between the speaker's intentions and the dynamics of conversation. Second, I have dealt with topic progression in general, and have tried to show that topic development may occur even when the interlocutors do not seem to have any specific intentions. In these cases, topic progression seems to come about according to a principle of neutral local coherence. Third, I have pointed to the difficulties of identifying speakers' intentions. Fourth, I have argued that any deviation from or violation of the principle of neutral local coherence may be taken as an indication of the existence of certain strategic, interactive or 'what for' intentions on the part of the violator. And last, I have discussed, briefly, emotionally induced violations which do not permit this intentional interpretation. Of similar interest are those cases in which the communicators do not seem either to have specific intentions or to be in a specific emotional state, but nevertheless behave as if they are aiming at specific goals. The examples discussed may be understood as instances of different forms of dynamics in dialogues, all of which deserve thorough further study.

References

Beach, W. A. (1983), 'Background understandings and the situated accomplishment of conversational telling-expansions', in R. T. Craig and K. Tracy (eds), *Conversational Coherence*, Beverly Hills and London: Sage.

Clark, H. H. and Schaefer, E. F. (1989), 'Collaborating on contributions to conversations', in R. Dietrich and C. F. Graumann (eds), *Language Processing in Social Context*, Amsterdam: North Holland.

Craig, R. T. and Tracy, K. (eds) (1983), *Conversational Coherence*, Beverly Hills and London: Sage.

Cranach, M. von (1986), 'Der Molch im Gewande oder Denken wir uns

eigentlich wirklich nichts bevor wir sprechen?' *Sprache und Kognition*, 5, 163–6.
Cranach, M. von, Kalbermatten, U., Indermühle, K. and Gugler, B. (1981), *Zielgerichtetes Handeln*, Bern: Huber.
Crow, B. K. (1983), 'Topic shifts in couples' conversations', in R. T. Craig and K. Tracy (eds), *Conversational Coherence*, Beverly Hills, Ca.: Sage.
Farrell, T. B. (1983), 'Aspects of coherence in conversation and rhetoric', in R. T. Craig and K. Tracy (eds), *Conversational Coherence*, Beverly Hills and London: Sage.
Foppa, K. (1978), 'Language acquisition – a humanethological problem?', *Social Science Information*, 17, 93–105.
Foppa, K. (1984), 'Redeabsicht und Verständigung', *Manuskripte*, 23, *Heft 84*, 73–6.
Foppa, K. (1987a), 'Dialogsteuerung', *Schweizerische Zeitschrift für Psychologie*, 46, 251–7.
Foppa, K. (1987b), '"Molche! Molche! Seid's gewesen!" (Frei nach J. W. Goethe)', *Sprache und Kognition*, 6, 41–4.
Foppa, K. (1987c), '"Richtige" oder "falsche" Empirie? Zum Problem der Rechtfertigung empirischer Verfahren in der Psychologie', in E. Raab and G. Schulter (eds), *Perspektiven psychologischer Forschung*, 3–12, Wien: Deuticke.
Foppa, K. and Käsermann, M. L. (1981), 'Das kindliche Wissen über Sprache: Ueberlegungen zu einem ungelösten Problem', in K. Foppa and R. Groner (eds), *Kognitive Strukturen und ihre Entwicklung*, Bern: Huber.
Graumann, C. F. (1989), 'Perspective setting and taking in verbal interaction', in R. Dietrich and C. F. Graumann (eds), *Language Processing in Social Context*, Amsterdam: North Holland.
Halisch, F. and Kuhl, J. (eds) (1987), *Motivation, Intention, and Volition*, Berlin: Springer.
Heritage, J. (1984), *Garfinkel and Ethnomethodology*, Cambridge: Polity Press.
James, W. (1890), *The Principles of Psychology*, New York: Holt.
Käsermann, M. L. (1980), *Spracherwerb und Interaktion*, Bern: Huber. (Ph.D dissertation University of Bern, 1978).
Käsermann, M. L. and Altorfer, A. (1989a), 'Family discourse: Physiological correlates of different degrees of stress', *British Journal of Psychiatry*, 155 (Suppl. 5), 136–43.
Käsermann, M. L. and Altorfer, A. (1989b), 'Obstruction in conversation: A triadic case study', *Journal of Language and Social Psychology*, 8, 49–58.
Käsermann, M. L. and Foppa, K. (1981), 'Some determinants of self correction: An interactional study of Swiss-German', in W. Deutsch (ed.), *The Child's Construction of Language*, London: Academic Press.
Kleist, H. von (1886–90), 'Ueber die allmähliche Verfertigung der Gedanken beim Reden', *Sämtliche Werke, Vierter Teil: Erzählungen, Vermischte Schriften*, ed. by T. Zolling.
Labov, W. and Fanshel, D. (1977), *Therapeutic Discourse: Psychotherapy as conversation*, New York: Academic Press.
Marková, I. (1987), 'On the interaction of opposites in psychological processes', *Journal for the Theory of Social Behaviour*, 17, 279–99.
Mead, G. H. (1934), *Mind, Self and Society*. Chicago, London: University of Chicago Press.

Moesch, K. (1987), *Prädikatzentrierte Einheiten als Basissegmente zur Analyse von Diskursen: ein pragmatischer Lösungsversuch*, unpublished manuscript, Bern.

Morawetz, A. and Walker, G. (1984), *Brief Therapy with Single-Parent Families*, New York: Brunner/Mazel.

Mühlemann, T. and Foppa, K. (1989), 'Simultansprechen und Sprecherwechsel', *Sprache und Kognition*, 8, 1–8.

Rommetveit, R. (1968), *Words, Meanings and Messages*, New York, London: Academic Press.

Schegloff, E. A. (1979), 'The relevance of repair to syntax for conversation', in T. Givón (ed.), *Syntax and Semantics*, New York: Academic Press.

Searle, J. R. (1969), *Speech Acts*, Cambridge: Cambridge University Press.

Wunderlich, D. (1976), *Studien zur Sprechakttheorie*, Frankfurt am Main: Suhrkamp.

9 | On the local sensitivity of conversation

Jörg R. Bergmann
Department of Sociology, University of Konstanz

Introduction

One of the most obvious 'dynamic' features of any kind of discourse is the topic development that takes place in and through the succeeding contributions to an ongoing verbal exchange. When talking, people always talk 'about something' and, although there are types of monotopic encounters, in most situations this 'something' does not remain the same as the interaction proceeds. Topic movement of some kind can be found within a single turn, as when a speaker, after finishing his or her story, draws a general conclusion. More often, however, topic development is an event which takes place across a series of turns and in which co-interactants find themselves talking about things that are quite different from the things they talked about a short time previously.

In this chapter I am going to consider a feature of topic talk that is of general relevance for any kind of verbal interaction, but that is most prominent in conversations and related types of discourse. The feature with which I shall be concerned materializes in those stretches of talk in which participants in a verbal exchange make an object or event in their immediate, witnessable environment the topic of their remarks. An instance of this kind of topicalization where *talk turns to local matters* can be found in the following excerpt taken from a family conversation.

I[1]
Family table talk about white collar crime and about a TV report on that issue

    A: then they u:h; (.) *sewed*–, then they:: .h sewed a *label* to it (0.5) saying 'Made by the People's Own Company So-and-so' and = put a label in and re-imported the very same shirts to the Federal Republic (0.5) because within the domestic trade in Germany, (.) you don't need to pay any duties, and = so
    U: uhu
                            (1 sec)
    A: A::::nd; that's how they made a killing;
                           (0.8)
→ *U*: °Look how the ⌈ cat is sleeping°
                       ⌊ (creaky noise)
→ *M*: I never saw her ⌈ lying like that;
→ *U*:   ⌊ (laughs]

(For a key to the symbols used in this and the following extracts see Atkinson and Heritage (1984, pp. ix–xvi).

Following A's description of a recent TV report on white collar crimes his sister U draws attention to the family's cat and its peculiar way of sleeping. M (who is A and U's mother) responds by confirming that the cat's position is most unusual. During the last part of her mother's utterance, U joins in with laughter.

When listening to recordings of family conversations, instances like the one just cited abound. That in talking to each other people turn to objects and events that are present in the situative context of their utterances is a regular recurring phenomenon that seems to be utterly trivial. During the various opportunities for talking in everyday life people comment on boundless things and events in the world; why shouldn't they attend in their talking to local objects and happenings as well? By itself, the simple fact that a verbal exchange turns to elements of its local environment seems to be most unremarkable. What else, then, makes this phenomenon a noteworthy object of analysis?

Some features of topic talk

Research during the last two decades has repeatedly shown that 'topic' is an extremely complex, multilayered discourse phenomenon that is not easily accessible to systematic investigation.[2] Any attempt to disentangle some of the components that the notion of topic incorporates will therefore be sketchy and selective. In this section I shall limit myself to a brief description of some of the main features of topic talk that are of relevance for the analysis which is to follow.

Topic progression

An initial characterization of the notion of topic can be obtained by singling out two complementary components which together form a contradictory unit. The first component may be conceived as the force that ensures that there is a topical flow at all. A verbal exchange that consists only of repetitions of the selfsame utterance and that therefore lacks any development would strike us as odd if not impossible (see Foppa, this volume, Chapter 8). There is a constraint of *progressivity* imposing on every speaker the obligation that in turn to talk he or she should be informative and should contribute something new to the ongoing verbal exchange.[3]

Topic maintenance

This component of topic progression is counterbalanced by a second feature. The demand for newness with which every speaker is faced cannot be met by just throwing in any 'new' item. There is a backward-oriented constraint on a speaker to stay on topic (Tracy, 1984), to adhere to the present subject matter and, more generally, to be concerned in the formulations he or she chooses with the 'co-selection of features for topic' (Schegloff, 1971, p. 95). It is part of a speaker's duties to show consideration for the maintenance of an actual topic and for the coherence of the unfolding discourse (Craig and Tracy, 1983). This is done preferably by shaping a single contribution to a verbal exchange in such a way that it is chained to another speaker's preceding utterance and adds something new to the actual topic which is thus sustained and continued. Speakers do, of course, make statements that are obviously produced out of topic. But these contributions are usually introduced by some kind of pre-positioned 'misplacement marker' (Schegloff and Sacks, 1973, p. 258), such as 'oh, by the way...', 'speaking of...' or 'not to change the topic but...'.[4] Through the use of these forms a speaker can display that he or she is well aware of the fact that his or her utterance is not topically coherent and is thus improperly placed. So, even when a speaker does not actually stay on topic he or she has ways of indicating his or her respect for the constraint of topicality.

Topic talk as joint production

There is a third organizational feature of topic talk that restricts a single participant's capacity to redirect the topic progression of a verbal exchange, in the same way as the obligation to stay on topic. A single utterance may by its form and content have the potential to lead to a change of topic. But whether such a change will in fact take place cannot be decided by the single actor alone, at least not in the case of verbal interaction.[5] Here, topic talk is a joint production and is dominated by the principle that 'it takes two to topic' (Covelli and Murray, 1980, p. 384). The direction into which the subject matter of a verbal exchange will develop is a socially negotiated accomplishment and does not depend simply on a single speaker's contribution. A topic move by one speaker may be supported or blocked, continued or transformed, assisted or ignored by his co-interactants and their response will influence the future progression of topic no less than the original utterance.

Topic formulations

The constraint to produce topically coherent contributions to an ongoing verbal exchange puts pressure on every participant to pay attention to the topic and the course it takes. Otherwise, participating in the talk may become difficult since every purported utterance will run the risk of not fitting the topic's actual state of development. This leads to a further relevant feature of topic talk: although interactants jointly orient to the topic of their exchange, what the topic consists of is by no means always formulated and put into words. Very often participants in a verbal exchange are busy talking without pinning a label on to their topic or announcing every single change in their topic orientation. Retrospectively, a verbal exchange may be described as 'a conversation about some eggheads in the department', even if this categorization did not actually occur in the conversation referred to. *Formulations* of topic[6] may be produced in the actual talk itself and may be seen as an attempt to ensure a shared understanding of what the talking is all about. But since topics develop further and since formulations are by their very nature glosses, meaning more than they can say in so many words, formulations of topic can provide only a momentary and tentative sense of orderliness and meaning for the participants.

Topic progression, topic maintenance, joint production of topic talk and topic formulations are but a few basic principles of the management of topic in verbal exchanges. They are not just analytic conceptions but features to which participants themselves are oriented in their actions. This will become evident in the rest of this chapter, which now turns to its main focus: the topicalization of local objects and events.

Topic, situation and the principle of local sensitivity

One of the most important general dimensions of social communication (as pointed out by Luckmann, this volume, Chapter 2) is 'abstraction', i.e. the ability of co-interactants to refer not only to components of the actual communicative situation but also to elements which transcend the situation in space or time. This faculty of abstraction by which people are capable of talking about things beyond the world within their reach is by no means self-evident. Clearly, new-born babies are perfectly able interactionally to synchronize their behaviour with other present persons, but they are, without any doubt, unable to communicate with others about some temporally or spatially remote object.[7] Studies in developmental pragmatics have further shown that, overwhelmingly, the conversations of young children are about objects, people or events that are present in the utterance context (Keenan and Schieffelin, 1976). The ability to expand the realm of possible topics beyond the immediate spatio-temporal environment of talking is the result of an ontogenetic development that has a phylogenetic parallel. According to Karl Bühler (1934/1965, pp. 366f.) the transition from basically 'empractical' acts of talking to 'independent, self-supplied speech products' is an act of liberation from situational aids (*'Situationshilfen'*) that must be seen as one of the most crucial factors in the development of human language.

The fact that participants in a verbal exchange have chosen as their topic some 'abstract' object outside of the encounter's situational surrounding does not imply that the talk produced is without any situational imprints. Utterances are never spoken out of context; they are always designed and shaped for specific recipients and are bound – particularly clearly in their deictic forms of reference – to extra-linguistic components of the situation. Language in use is essentially indexical (Garfinkel and Sacks, 1970), which is to say that participants in verbal exchanges are sensitive to context, and this holds true even if the subject matter of talk is not to be found within the situational environment of the talking itself.

Adult humans are equipped with the capability to focus their verbal exchanges on abstract – in the sense of extra-situational – objects and at the same time to show in their utterances an orientation towards situational particulars. This observation leads to the heart of the matter. Obviously, a basic feature of the communicative competence of human beings is their ability to split attention in such a way that they can simultaneously deal with objects-at-a-distance (topics) and attend to objects-within-reach (local matters). In telling a story about a past event (and thereby concentrating on an object that transcends the situation) a speaker does not shut off his or her eyes, ears and nose, but remains alert to whatever is going on within his or her sphere of perception. An even stronger split of attention may be found in those cases in which a person participates in a conversation and at the same time is occupied with knitting or some other manual activity. A crucial question arises at this point: how are these two domains of attention related? Do they conflict with each other?[8] Is one of them basically subordinated to the other? Or is there a dynamic hierarchization by which each domain in turn may, for a while, be the dominant one?

I suggest that in every kind of discourse there operates a basic principle which I shall call the principle of 'local sensitivity' and which can be described as the structural tendency built into every topic talk to turn to local matters. This description needs further qualification since it is evident that the term 'local matters' can mean two things. First, at any given moment in the course of a verbal exchange the talk so far and especially the immediately prior utterance can be regarded as the 'local environment' in which every next turn must position itself and to which it must adapt. This notion of 'local', which is the common one in conversation analysis,[9] refers to the talk-so-far-as-the-condition-for-every-next-turn and may incorporate sequential implications, the constraint to stay on topic, etc. But there is another, an extra-linguistic notion of 'local' as well. The talk-so-far does not make up the entire 'local environment' in which a next turn has to be placed. There are matters outside of the verbal flow itself – objects at hand and situative events – which can be perceived by the actors and which in themselves constitute a separate local context for next actions.

It is this second notion of local that I have in mind when I speak of 'local sensitivity'. Thus, the concept of local sensitivity is introduced not to refer to the sequential and topical conditions for any next turn, but instead to the present extra-verbal, situational locale in which a next utterance gets placed and realized. Local sensitivity is meant to capture the tendency built into every topic talk to focus on elements of the encounter's context which are situated or occur in the participants' field of perception but have not been topicalized so far.

Since every discoursive process is situationally embedded, it is possible in every discourse to (re-)focus on components of its local environment and make them the topic of the verbal exchange. However, various types of discourse differ significantly in the degree to which their topic progression is subject to the principle of local sensitivity. This may even be seen as an identifying feature of discourse types, providing each of them with their distinctive character of higher or lesser local sensitivity.

Turning to local matters

The easiest way to observe the principle of local sensitivity in operation is to examine those occasions where in the course of a verbal exchange some object within the participants' field of perception 'imposes' its relevance (Schutz and Luckmann, 1973/1974, pp. 186–90) onto the interactants. An unknown object, a strange sound, a funny smell, a long expected (or surprising) arrival may capture the actors' attention, thus drawing it away from whatever it is presently directed at. Very frequently it can be observed that these events not only lead to a restructuring of the participants' attention but to a change in topic as well. Talk about the previous topic stops and the verbal exchange focuses instead on the intruding object. This happens in example II.

II[10]

    A: ⎡ Branko Zebesch must have been drunk (0.5)
        ⎣ again;
    W: During the week he is sober for three days;
    A: (Laughs)
    HJ: What?
               (3.0)
    W: And his friends and patrons say of him that in those three days during the week when he is sober; he achieves more than many a coach who is sober for seven days;
               (3.0)

```
              (Hugo, the budgerigar, comes flying into the room)
  ←   A:   (towards Hugo) Hallo there;
                            (1.0)
  ←   U:   (towards Hugo) Hallo = Hallo there
                            (2.0)
  ←   U:   (towards Hugo) Come here (0.5) come!
  ←   A:   (towards Hugo) Come on look
      U:   Is there any water left?
      A:   It's all gone
  →  HJ:   But a bird like that for sure is not a gourmet;
      H:   Huh?
  →  HJ:   I said a bird like that for sure is not a gourmet
  →   H:   (Given that it is always) eating grain
                            (4.0)
  →   H:   ⎡ It's just all the time on a grain diet
  →   U:   ⎣ hm – sometimes it eats croissants;
```

In this instance the members of a family are talking about a well-known football coach and his publicly reported problems with alcohol when the family's budgerigar makes its appearance by flying across the family table. The bird is addressed and lured immediately by some of the family members (marked by the symbol ←). After some attempts the interactants stop directing their remarks to the budgerigar and start commenting about it instead (marked by the symbol →). In the ensuing talk, this pattern whereby utterances addressed *to* the bird are continued by comments and stories *about* it, recurs.

The noise of a car accident, or just the rumble given by a co-participant's stomach, the sun blinking suddenly through the clouds, or just the cat's peculiar sleeping position, a smell of smoke, or just a waft of perfume – whatever it is in the local environment of an encounter that attracts the interactants' attention, it can also be turned into a topic of talk. However, the principle of local sensitivity can be found in operation not only in those instances where some conspicuous object or event intrudes and draws the participants' attention, and subsequently the topic of their talk, away from their present involvement. As can be seen in the following data segment, participants in a conversation may also topicalize objects within their field of perception that by no means impose themselves, but are just there in the situation (and have been all along).

III[11]
    J: Oh I could drive if you want me to.
    C: Well no I'll drive (I don' m⌈in')
    J: ⌊hhh
               (1.0)
    J: I mea*nt* to offah.
              (16.0)
→ *J*: Those shoes look nice when you keep on putting stuff on 'em.
    C: Yeah I 'ave to get another can cuz cuz it ran out.
        I mean it's a⌈lmost (h) ou(h)*t=
    J: ⌊Oh:::ah*he .hh heh=
    C: =yeah well it cleans 'em and keeps⌈'em clean.
    J: ⌊Yeah right=
    C: =I should get a brush too and *you* should getta brush'n
       ⌈*you* should–* fix your hiking boo⌈ts
    J: ⌊yeah suh::   ⌊my hiking boots
    C: which you were gonna do this weekend.
    J: Pooh, did I have time this wk– well::
    C: Ahh c'mon=
    J: =wh'n we get– (uh::kay), I haven't even sat down to do any– y'know like .hh today I'm gonna sit down 'n read while you're doing yur coat, (0.7) do yur– hood.
    C: Yehhh=
    J: =(ok) (2.0) I haven't *not* done *any*thing the whole *week*end.
    C: (okay)
              (14.0)
→ *J*: Dass a rilly nice swe::der, (.hh) 'at's my favorite sweater on you, it's the only one that looks right on you.
    C: mm huh.
              (90.0)
       (Sacks, Schegloff and Jefferson, 1974, pp. 714f.)

It was not J's shoes and sweater that made the topic change by attracting C's attention. It was C who, out of the multitude of possible things in the world to talk about, selected and raised those 'sleeping' objects in the participants' environment and who, by commenting on those objects, made them the topic of talk.

Whether participants in a verbal exchange start to topicalize elements or events in their immediately perceptible environment does not depend solely on the force with which these objects intrude into the perceptual field of an actor. The street noise that is to be heard in an apartment can be turned into a topic of talk – but so can the absence of any street noise. Of course, an unfamiliar object 'draws' the actors' attention to itself by its very unfamiliarity (and so do other surprising or obtrusive events). But the barking of a dog or a conspicuous dirty mark on a co-participant's shirt can also be ignored – and very often must be ignored – by an actor. It is therefore always the interactants themselves who in a given situation allow the principle of local sensitivity to determine the flow and change of topic. As always, however, people cannot just do whatever they want. Whether the topic in a verbal exchange can shift to situational objects is not just a matter of personal choice. There are types of discourse in which the principle of local sensitivity is tightly controlled, and others in which participants are to a high degree permitted to turn – in their attention as well as in their talking – to local matters.

Local sensitivity as an organizational feature of conversation

A discourse type particularly suitable for the study of how and where an ongoing course of verbal interaction is shaped by the principle of local sensitivity is conversation. It is within conversation that a participant may change topic by, for example, commenting on an ashtray he or she is using, by asking about some visible gadget that arouses his or her interest, or by pointing out the peculiar behaviour of a pet. This observation would be quite unremarkable if it were simply the case that the situational environment of a verbal exchange is accessible to 'conversation' – as a thematic field – but off limits to other types of discourse. But the matter is more interesting than that. The possibility of topicalizing local matters is, rather, part of the social organization of conversational interaction and closely related to its other features (see Adato, 1980). Some of these features will be recalled shortly in order to underline the significance that the principle of local sensitivity has for the organization of conversation.

Conversational interaction is characterized, among other things, by the fact that it is not restricted to a single recurrent interactional pattern, such as the question–answer sequence in interviews, or the question–answer–evaluation sequence classroom interaction. Instead, there is a kaleidoscope of social activities (telling jokes, teasing, arguing, teaching, gossiping, etc.) that may occur and shape its course. Furthermore, the flow of interaction is not fixed in advance by formal regulation, an agenda or liturgy. It emerges turn by turn. In the same way, topic progression in conversation is not predetermined but is usually achieved gradually, by stepwise transition in which one topic flows into another without interactants noticing.[12]

As these features show, conversations are far less tightly bound than other types of discourse by a corset of formal patterns of interaction. Conversations are also far less constricted by thematic bonds originating in the given purpose of an encounter and narrowing the directions of progression. But there is another side to this freedom. Because conversations are not backed up by formal procedural rules, because they are not guided by a developmental scheme and are not kept on a thematic leash they may 'get into trouble'. Transcripts of conversations reveal that very often the self-organizing power of conversation temporally decreases, remarks are not taken up by recipients and are left without comment, a topic dries up without a new topic emerging, periods of silence become more frequent, the overall conversation is in danger of petering out. In an interview, the interviewer would pose the next question; in a business meeting, the chairperson would move to the next item on the agenda. But conversations live on the 'endogenous' production and continuation of topics, for which every competent participant can be held responsible. Since 'conversation' is based on the voluntary commitment of all participants, an increasing number of periods of silence may imply that a closing phase is approaching. They indicate that there is nothing more to talk about and hence no point in staying together any longer.[13] If there is nothing left that participants want to tell each other, they may decide that they might as well depart.

In situations like these, where talk becomes discontinuous and gets stuck in a period of slackness, the possibility of topicalizing objects and events in the local environment is an important resource to ensure the continuation of interaction. Of course, participants in a conversation talk mainly about 'abstract' things beyond the encounter's immediate local context. They argue about Stalingrad or Boris Becker, they imagine a future wedding or jointly remember last year's holiday trip, they tell each other how to ride a bus without paying and they make fun of a distant relative. But as soon as the verbal flow stops, the topic line along which a conversation proceeds is cut off. Given that the old topic line has already come to a closure, a special effort involving the giving of a reason for reopening the conversation would be necessary to pick it up again. In order to start the conversation anew one may instead refer to some element or event within the perceptual field of all participants. Relying in such a situation on the principle of local sensitivity has various advantages.

It is part of our everyday experience that talk that initially focuses on an object in the participants' immediate presence very quickly moves on from there to quite different topics. An example of such a rapid topical shift is provided in the following segment.

IV[14]
Family sitting at the dinner table, starting to eat

```
W:      Enjoy your meal!
                                    (1.0)
HJ:     Enjoy ⌈ your meal!
U:            ⌊ Enjoy your meal!
                                    (3.0)
A:      Enjoy your meal!
                                    (2.0)
U:      M:::, quite garlicky
HJ:     Is it?
                                    (6.0)
        Well;=°no one could taste it at all yesterday°
        °°(         )°°
                                    (3.0)
U:      M:::, these little carrots are delicious;
                                    (3.0)
A:      °°(         )°°
                                    (6.0)
U:      Oh dear, mum; (0.5) the amount of carrots I eat, I should have
        very good eyes by now;
                                    (3.0)
        all fresh ones;
                                    (5.0)
U:      °I got a prescription for new glasses;°
        I mean just the lenses.
                                    (3.0)
A:      you kept the old frame, didn't you Uschi.
U:      Yeah of course
                                    (2.5)
H:      With Karin's glasses, (0.5) she wanted to have new frames, =
        but they're not available any more, (.) and on her old glasses (.)
        the colour's peeling off; (1.0) and as she really wanted to have
        the same ones and the same ones weren't available any longer
        as I said; (1.0) the optician suggested to her that she should
        get the colour and then they could be resprayed;
HJ:     Ye ⌈ ah,
A:         ⌊ Uhu:,
```

In this extract conversation moves from a first comment about the meal ('quite garlicky') to a second remark about another food component (carrots) and from there – via the implicit proposition that carrots are good for the eyes – to information about a prescription for new glasses and then to a story about a woman who was going to get the frames of her glasses renewed in an unusual way. As can be seen in this instance, talk about some local object or event – dinner table conversations with all their empractical activities being a good case in point[15] – may serve as a kind of 'trigger topic'. Thus the ongoing conversation may be shifted quickly to a topic that was hitherto unthought of and that transcends the immediate situation.[16]

The principle of local sensitivity may be used by the participants especially in cases of discontinuous talk as a 'first gear' to set a conversation that has come to a halt in motion again. Those specific conversational circumstances that Schegloff and Sacks (1973, p. 262) have called a 'continuing state of incipient talk' – they have in mind 'members of a household in their living room, employees who share an office, passengers together in an automobile, etc.' (*ibid.*) – provide fertile ground for local topicalization after a temporary halt of topical progression. It is the kind of 'environment' in which people know that they will share one another's presence for a certain time and in which chunks of talk alternate with long periods of silence. These silences are not seen by the co-participants as leading to a definitive termination of talk. None the less, a restart of the verbal exchange is usually not possible simply by 'continuing' the discontinued previous topic line. On occasions like these, participants may choose instead to recommence talking by directing recipients' attention to an object or event in the situational here and now, trusting that a short-range remark will soon trigger off talk on more remote objects.

Topicalizing a local object may be used as a device not only to recommence a discontinued verbal exchange within a conversation but also to initiate a conversation itself. Time and again, conversations between strangers have been started by some remark on the weather, on the slowness of a train, or on the (good or poor) quality of a certain dish.[17] Referring to local matters can function as a topic initiation because the way this activity is organized provides a solution to a structural problem of topic talk. Making reference to an object or event within an encounter's local environment is a topical mechanism that is capable of answering a question which for participants in a verbal exchange is a pervasively relevant issue: the question of placement. In producing or hearing an utterance, conversationalists are continuously concerned with the question of 'why that now?' (Schegloff and Sacks, 1973, p. 241; for some further differentiations see Bilmes, 1985). That is to say, co-interactants take the verbal exchange immediately preceding an utterance as an interpretative resource by which an understanding of what that utterance was all about can be reached.

At the very beginning of a conversation, or after a long period of silence, no sequential environment is available that could be considered by the interlocutors to explain the occurrence of any utterance. In such circumstances every utterance is, so to speak, placed out of the sequential context which is usually provided by the talk thus far; an important source of understanding is therefore missing. By focusing on a local object or event a speaker invites his or her hearers to draw upon their perceptual awareness in order to identify what he or she is talking about. The speaker thereby not only invokes the perceivable extra-verbal environment as the relevant context of his or her utterance, but also enables his or her hearers to take their own perceptions as a source by which a solution to the placement question may be arrived at. For example, a recipient who sees with his or her own eyes the peculiar sleeping posture of a cat is also able to recognize why his or her attention and the conversation's topic was directed to it by the speaker.

There are further, deeper connections between the principle of local sensitivity and the social organization of conversation as a specific type of discourse, than their usefulness for opening up or restarting verbal exchange. In his famous essay on 'sociability' Georg Simmel showed that:

> conversation cannot allow any content to become significant in its own right. As soon as the discussion becomes objective [*sachlich*], as soon as it makes the ascertainment of a truth its *purpose*, it ceases to be sociable and thus becomes untrue to its own nature. (Simmel, 1917/1950, p. 62)[18]

Transcripts of family conversations reveal, however, that despite Simmel's statement, conversations are frequently in danger of becoming 'objective' and of degenerating even into potentially serious quarrels. One reason for this is that on the one hand disagreements are necessary as the communicative activity that keeps conversations alive, while on the other hand disagreements, by their very social organization, may lead to blocking of the topic or tend to escalate. In such a situation the principle option of shifting attention to local objects and topicalizing local events can serve as an effective antidote.

Any type of discourse that submits to the principle of local sensitivity is almost bound to be subject to rapid and unforeseeable topic shifts. By turning from what is actually talked about to a local event and by virtue of the above-mentioned trigger effect of talk about local objects, the progression of topic – and hence the abandonment of old topics – can be dramatically accelerated. Given this capacity, the principle of local sensitivity can be used whenever, during conversation, a discussion becomes too objective, a disagreement loses its playful character or a topic tends to drag on unduly. 'The ability to change topics easily and quickly is part of the nature of sociable conversation', stated Simmel (1917/1950, p. 63). The principle of local sensitivity is a major component of the social organization of conversation by which this characteristic is brought about and maintained.

When co-interactants turn, in their talking, to local matters, they orient their talk towards components of the communicative situation which are simultaneously accessible to both of them. A remark on the weather may thus not only change the topic of talk but also its 'footing' (Goffman, 1979) by invoking situational circumstances to which both co-participants are exposed in the same way. By directing attention to local matters, co-participants abandon, at least for a short moment, their participatory roles deriving from extra-situational bonds and take on a shared situation identity of being e.g. a 'witness' or a 'victim' of a local event.[19] As talk moves on, this co-membership may, of course, soon be abandoned again in favour of other relational identities. But for a short moment mediated by the shared experience of some local event, there was a sense of mutuality, a realization of 'the synchronism of two streams of consciousness' (Schutz, 1967, p. 102) that joined the co-participants together. Thus, the principle of local sensitivity always implies a moment of 'phatic communion' (Malinowski, 1946). This may be a major reason why this feature of topic management is so densely interwoven with the social organization of conversation.

Controlling local sensitivity

I have portrayed conversation as a type of discourse whose topical organization is forcefully characterized by the principle of local sensitivity. This description is warranted by the fact that, in contrast to other types of discourse, conversation can include two anarchic types of participants: small children and pets.[20] By their way of behaving they often draw the 'ordinary' interlocutor's attention to local matters. It would be insufficient, however, to view conversation as a type of encounter that can tolerate the anomic and unpredictable activities of these 'participants'. This is merely an aspect of a more generally important feature of this discourse type which is the fact that in order to maintain its flow conversation can systematically capitalize on the impulsive way of acting of children and pets by turning them into the topic of talk.

It is even possible to single out some types of conversational groups whose topic talk is almost entirely based on the principle of local sensitivity. These groups are organized in such a way that the distraction of the group members' attention and the shift of topic talk induced by local events is not inhibited but facilitated. In a classical ethnographic study of a small American rural community (West – pseud. for C. Withers – 1945) one can find a description of a 'loafing group', consisting of old men who spend most of their time exchanging stories and gossip, while sitting on two iron benches in one corner of the square. 'The iron benches control a view of the street and everyone who enters it from any direction. The Old Men daily gather up all threads of current events and gossip' (*ibid.*, pp. 99ff).[21] As can be seen from their specific micro-ecological arrangement, gossip groups of this kind are focused on and strongly dependent upon local events which are immediately turned into 'topical fuel' in order to keep the 'conversational apparatus' running.[22] In these cases, local sensitivity is a dominating feature of talk. But at the other polar extreme, there are types of discourse in which the principle of local sensitivity is tightly controlled.

At the entrance to churches, courthouses or universities, visitors are usually reminded by a special sign that it is prohibited to take pets into those areas. (Similarly, attending a lecture or seminar together with one's small children is, although there is no written notice, mostly regarded as a violation of proper academic behaviour.) Such regulations directly concern the question of how the issue of local sensitivity is handled in official discourse within these types of institution. It is a characteristic feature of institutional discourse types such as courtroom proceedings, seminar sessions or doctor–patient interactions that co-participants are acting under the constraint to orient themselves towards the official, predefined goal of the encounter. Precisely because of its goal- and task-oriented character, institutional discourse is continuously faced with the danger of distraction.

A major source of distraction is, of course, the local, situational environment of these institutional encounters. During a seminar session a helicopter may land just outside the university building; during a wedding ceremony a participant who has fallen asleep may begin to snore; during a courtroom proceeding a window cleaner may start to do his job. In these situations participants usually feel obliged to disregard the intruding events, that is to say, to control the urge arising from the principle of local sensitivity and concentrate on the matter at hand. But many of them may nevertheless covertly watch the obtrusive happening, while simultaneously pretending to remain faithful to the official topic. At this point it becomes apparent that there is in fact a tendency built into every conversation or, more generally, discourse, to focus on elements of the encounter's context which are situated or occur in the participants' field of perception.

It is a general feature of institutional discourse that it remains insensitive to local matters, which means that the principle of local sensitivity must be controlled. Topic talk in institutional discourse may only turn to local matters in cases of perceivable emergency or in cases of obvious emergency in which some circumstances or happenings make continuation of the institutional discourse impossible. An experience that one can have again and again (e.g. in seminar sessions) is that, once the control of local sensitivity in institutional discourse is relaxed due to some interfering event, participants immediately turn to all sorts of local business and it usually needs several restarts and admonitions before they are tuned in again on the official agenda.

The problem of staying on topic in institutional discourse could, of course, be solved by putting all the burden on the participants and holding them responsible for the effective control of local sensitivity. But it is obviously only to a limited extent that people can prevent themselves from turning to local matters when things happen within their field of perception. A manifestation of this can be found in the fact that institutions themselves take precautions against possible distractions resulting from local irritations, e.g by keeping away children and pets. This may be the meaning of ceremonial regulations within institutions in general – they are there to maintain the situation as defined, i.e. the official topic of the encounter, by preventing the participants' attention from wandering to the bewildering array of diversions presented by the principle of local sensitivity.

Local sensitivity and the 'naturalness' of conversational data: a methodological afterthought

In this concluding section I shall show how the argument I have presented in this chapter has a methodological bearing on studies that deal with 'natural' data. In recent years it has become increasingly fashionable for sociological, linguistic and psychological research to use audiotapes, videotapes and transcripts of naturally occurring interactions as primary data.[23] Interactions may be regarded as 'naturally occurring' insofar as they are not elicited by a researcher, i.e. are not artifically produced in an experiment or interview, but are happening anyway in and as a real-life event. During the process of data collection, researchers working with 'natural' data find themselves in the position of having to decide whether they should deceive or inform the interactants about the fact that their behaviour will be continuously recorded. (Given the bulkiness – and visibility – of the equipment, this question is mostly irrelevant in the case of video recordings.)

In order to avoid the ethical problems that must be faced when people are recorded without their prior consent, many researchers opt to switch on the recorder only after they have notified those whose behaviour they want to document. But this solution may lead to the very same problem which researchers encounter when they use experimental or survey data and which motivated them to focus instead on 'naturally' occurring interaction in the first place: once people have been informed that they will be recorded, their awareness of that fact influences their behaviour. In his essay on the sociology of the secret, Simmel pointed out the importance and consequentiality of the fact that 'no other object of knowledge than man modifies its behavior in view of the fact that it is aware of being observed' (Simmel, 1908 p. 258). What direction this modification will take is hard to tell. How an actor's awareness of him- or herself as an object of observation may influence his or her actual behaviour varies from one individual to another. In any case it is also an unwelcome circumstance to the researcher who has shifted to 'naturally' occurring interaction as a source of his data to avoid the methodological limitations of experimental and survey data.[24] A common strategy used by many researchers to rescue the 'naturalness' of their data is to instruct the interactants who have been selected for observation to act as naturally as possible and simply to disregard and ignore the presence of the camera and/or microphone. The non-occurrence of any remark about the recording situation is then seen as evidence that the interactants did indeed forget that they were being recorded, and on the basis of this lack of comment, the data are deemed to be natural.

The paradoxicality of the instruction to act naturally and to disregard the recording situation can be fully appreciated once the feature of local sensitivity is taken into account. In the case of discourse types that are characterized by tight control of topic progression and that protect themselves – often by means of ritualization – against possible digressions induced by local events, the awareness of being observed and recorded does not seem to have a strong effect on the actors' actual behaviour. Participants in a scientific debate, in a courtroom proceeding or in a wedding ceremony know that their behaviour will be scrutinized by a critical opponent, a suspicious adversary or a curious public audience. These actors are therefore already under some 'natural' surveillance, to which the presence of a recording machine as a further observational tool would not add significantly. Instructing them to act as 'naturally' as possible in front of a camera would be futile, since for them the constraint of acting as if in front of a camera is part of the 'naturalness' of the scene itself.

However, as soon as the researcher moves backstage with his or her recording equipment, the situation changes entirely. In the case of discourse types that are characterized by informality, casualness and privacy, the participants' awareness of being observed and recorded may heavily affect their actual behaviour. This is in part due to the fact that words spoken in private are usually produced and looked on as elements of an 'unplanned discourse' (Ochs, 1979) and are therefore quite unprotected and vulnerable, and demand confidentiality and benevolent understanding. This is no longer guaranteed once those words, spoken in private, are on record.

Given that social behaviour in informal, sociable situations are particularly susceptible to the actors' awareness of being an object of observation and recording, how should a researcher proceed? He or she might be inclined to notify his or her subjects of the recording, and to urge them not to pay any attention to it during their interaction. But such an instruction, although generated by the motive of keeping the interaction as natural as possible, would lead to a particularly *un*natural situation. It is a constitutive feature of interactional systems of this kind that they are to a very high degree locally sensitive and allow for the possibility of topicalizing objects and events within their situational environment. It is therefore the most 'natural' thing for interactants who know that their conversation is recorded, to comment on the recording itself.

The twofold instruction to act naturally and to ignore the recording situation is thus, at least with regard to conversations and other types of informal discourse, deeply paradoxical. Contrary to the general opinion of many social researchers who work with 'natural' data, I would argue that if recordings of naturally occurring informal interactions do not contain any part during which the participants make reference to the fact that they are being recorded, then this absence is conspicuous and can be taken to be a reliable sign of the '*un*naturalness' of the documented interaction.

Appendix: Original German transcripts

Extract I

Familiengespräch, über organisiertes Verbrechen, Wirtschaftskriminalität und eine Fernsehsendung über dieses Thema

A: hen so do: a:; (.) Zettl, neih– hen se::
.h oba: neignäh:t, (0.5) gefertigd von Vau E Be:
Soundso::, und=an Zettl neiglegd und die gleiche
Hemda; .h wieder in d'Bundesrepublik; eigfüh:rd
(0.5) weil: im innerdeutscha Handel, (.) brauchsch
koine Zölle za::hla, und=so
U: mhm
(1.0)
A: Un::::d; so hen die:, da Riesa Reibach gmachd;
(0.8)
U: °Guck mal wie die ⎡ Katze schloaft°
⎣ (*knarrende Geräusche*)
M: So han 'se no nie ⎡ liega säha;
U: ⎣ (*lacht*)

Extract II

A: Na der Branko Zebesch muß ja wieder besoffn (0.5)
gwesen sein;
W: Drei Tage in der Woche isser nüchtern;
A: (*lacht*)
HJ: Was?
(3.0)
W: Und sein Freund und Gönner sagen ihm nach
daß er in drei Tagen in der Woche nüchtern;
mehr erreicht als mancher Trainer der auch sieben
Tage nüchtern is;
(3.0)
(*Hugo, der Wellensittich, kommt ins Zimmer geflogen*)
A: (*zu Hugo*) Grüß Gott;
(1.0)

U: (*zu Hugo*) Grüß Gott=Grüß Gott
(2.0)
U: (*zu Hugo*) Komm her (0.5) komm
A: (*zu Hugo*) paß mal auf
U: Gibt's Wasser,
A: Alles weg
HJ: Aber a Gurmee is so a Vogel wirklich ne;
H: Hm?
HJ: Ich sag a Gurmee is so a Vogel wirklich ne
H: (Wenn er immer) Körner frißt
(4.0)
H: ⎡ Der macht halt immer ne Körnerkur
U: ⎣ hm (–) dr frißt mal Kroasoo;

Extract IV

Die Familie sitzt am Tisch und beginnt mit dem Essen
W: Mahlzeit!
(1.0)
HJ: Mahl ⎡ zeit!
U: ⎣ Mahlzeit!
(3.0)
A: Mahlzeit!
(2.0)
U: No, gud knoblauchig;
HJ: Ja:?
(6.0)
Naja;=°nachdem mr gestern nischt davon geschmeckt hat° °°(   )°°
(3.0)
U: M:::, sind die Möhrlen gud;
(3.0)
A: °°(   )°°
(6.0)
U: Oje Mamma; (0.5) da müsst ja ich schon sehr gutte Augen ham=was ich manchmal Möhren ess;
(3.0)
alles frische;
(5.0)
U: °Ich hab mirne neue Brille verschreiben lassen;°
neue Gläser halt.
(3.0)

A: in die alte Fassung 'nein, Uschi ja,
U: ja freilich
(2.5)
H: bei dr Karin ihrer Brille, (0.5) die wollte
a neues Gestell habn, =des gibts aber nimmer,
(.) weil bei der alten Brille, (.) der Lack
abgeblättert isch; (1.0) und nachdem s' dann
unbedingt wieder die gleiche habn wollte, =und
's die gleiche wieg'sagt nimmer gibt, (1.0)
hat jetzt der Optiker gsagt sie soll den Lack
besorgen, und dann wird se umgespritzt;
HJ: J ⌈ a,
A: ⌊ mhm:,

Notes

1. English translation of a German conversation. The original German transcript segments can be found in the Appendix.
2. Studies that introduce the concept of topic within an interactional perspective can be found in Keenan and Schieffelin (1976) and in Gumperz, Aulakh and Kaltman (1982). For a recent description of studies in the field of conversation analysis that deal with topical organization, see Heritage (1985).
3. With regard to sequential organization, Schegloff (1979, p. 269 fn) speaks of a 'general preference for "progressivity", that is, for "next parts" of structured units (e.g. turns, turn-constructional units like sentences, stories, etc.) to come next'.
4. See Planalp and Tracy (1980). Goffman (1976, p. 18) refers to these hedged self-reflective comments as 'weak bridges'. Digressions (see Dascal and Katriel, 1979) must be distinguished from encapsulated 'side sequences' (see Jefferson, 1972) after which topic talk is resumed.
5. Someone who is giving a lecture or writing a paper faces a different situation. Within the limits of a predefined subject he or she has got much more freedom to decide by him- or herself the direction in which the topic of his or her text will move.
6. In the meaning developed by Garfinkel and Sacks (1970, p. 350) and described by them in the following way:
   A member may treat some part of the conversation as an occasion to describe that conversation, to explain it, or characterize it, or furnish the gist of it, or take note of its accordance with rules, or remark on its departure from rules. That is to say, a member may use some part of the conversation as an occasion to *formulate* the conversation.
The concept of 'formulation' was further elaborated by Heritage and Watson (1979), who were able to show that formulations, by virtue of their 'fixing' a conversation's topic, help to render conversations preservable and reportable. That formulations of topic in an institutional setting may turn into a source of trouble is nicely shown in a study of classroom talk by Heyman (1986).

7. See e.g. the research by Trevarthen and Hubley (1978).
8. I remember quite vividly the heated discussions at German universities some years ago when quite a few – male as well as female – students regularly insisted on knitting during seminar sessions.
9. See Sacks, Schegloff and Jefferson (1974, p. 725). There the turn-taking system for conversation is characterized by the authors as the 'local management system, in that all the operations are "local", i.e. directed to "next turn" and "next transition" on a turn-by-turn basis.' Allocation of turns and turn-size are 'accomplished locally, i.e. in the developmental course of each turn, under constraints imposed by a next turn, and by an orientation to a next turn in the current one' (*ibid.*).
10. English translation of a German conversation. The original German transcript segments can be found in the Appendix.
11. In Sacks, Schegloff and Jefferson (1974) this data segment is quoted in order to show that lapses occur in an ongoing conversation which can thus be discontinuous.
12. See Harvey Sacks' pioneering remarks on topic management in his lectures of 1967 and 1968. Jefferson (1984) shows for a certain interactional environment (the continuation of a conversation after talk about a trouble) that co-interactants may have to use some delicate methods to manage this stepwise transition from one topic to another. Despite this preference for stepwise transition, participants in a conversation also use specific topic initial elicitors as is shown by Button and Casey (1984) and Wilson (1987).
13. On the closing-implicative meaning of silences, see Maynard (1980). How, in situations like these, talk can nevertheless be continued is analysed by Button (1987). Luhmann (1975) argues that the occurrence of silences immediately endangers the maintenance of an elementary social system, such as a conversation, that is constituted by mutual perceptibility.
14. English translation of a German conversation. The original German transcript segments can be found in the Appendix.
15. It is not by chance therefore that a dinner table conversation is the object of analysis in a paper by Erickson (1982, p. 45) that deals with the social construction of topical cohesion through the combination of 'three types of production resources that conversationalists can make use of: "immediately local" resources, "local resources once removed" from the immediate scene, and "nonlocal" resources.' And in a paper in which 'displaced and situated language' are systematically distinguished as two separate pragmatic modes, Auer (1988) also uses an excerpt taken from a dinner conversation to demonstrate his point.
16. With reference to a distinction introduced by Jefferson (1984, p. 221), remarks about local objects and events may be regarded as constituting a topic type that is 'open' to immediate introduction of any next topic, whereas e.g. a troubles-telling is topically 'closed' in that it constrains what sort of talk should properly come next.
17. These initiating remarks on local matters very often seem to be made in the format of first assessments which provide the relevance of second assessments to be produced by the recipients (see Pomerantz, 1984). How these initiating assessments, by the way they are shaped, exploit the preference organization operating with respect to assessments, such that topical shifts to non-local objects in the subsequent talk are facilitated, is a question beyond consideration in this paper.

18. I have taken the liberty of changing the available English translation of Simmel's text on the basis of the German original.
19. It can be observed that people who are mutual strangers and who would never exchange greetings when they meet each other on the street in their home city, do exchange greetings (often without making any further remarks) when they meet as mountain hikers. There they share the same situated identity as hikers which is derived from the spatio–temporal surrounding of their encounter and in which they relate to each other. The exchange of greetings is thus a recognition and acknowledgement of co-membership derived from the encounter's local environment.
20. See my paper on pets as communicative resources (Bergmann, 1988), that is in many respects complementary to this chapter on local sensitivity.
21. A similar description can be found in Wylie's (1957) ethnography of a village in the Vaucluse. In this case it is a group of housewives who met daily in a corner of the village square just opposite the café 'which was a strategic place because everybody had to go past it. A more general treatment of gossip groups and their local sensitivity can be found in my book on gossip as a communicative genre (Bergmann, 1987, pp. 102f.).
22. On the concept of 'conversational apparatus' and its functions within intimate social relationships, see Berger and Kellner (1964/1970, p. 61).
23. For some crucial epistemological implications of recordings as data in interpretive sociology and for a critique of some of the ways in which data of this kind are used in social science research, see Bergmann (1985).
24. Textbooks on social research methods deal with this phenomenon under various labels, such as: demand characteristics, social acceptability of answers in questionnaires etc.

References

Adato, A. (1980). '"Occasionality" as a constituent feature of the known-in-common character of topics'. *Human Studies*, 3, 47–64.

Atkinson, J. M. and Heritage, J. (eds) (1984), *Structures of Social Action: Studies in conversation analysis*, Cambridge: Cambridge University Press.

Auer, P. (1988), 'On deixis and displacement', *Folia Linguistica*, 22, 263–92.

Berger, P. L. and Kellner, H. (1964/1970), 'Marriage and the construction of reality: An exercise in the microsociology of knowledge', *Diogenes* 46, reprinted in H. P. Dreitzel (ed.), *Recent Sociology, no. 2*, New York: The Macmillan Co.; London: Collier-Macmillan, 1970.

Bergmann, J. R. (1985), 'Flüchtigkeit und methodische Fixierung sozialer Wirklichkeit: Aufzeichnungen als Daten der interpretativen Soziologie', in W. Bonss and H. Hartmann (eds), *Entzauberte Wissenschaft* (Sonderband 3 der *Sozialen Welt*), Göttingen: Otto Schwartz.

Bergmann, J. R. (1987), *Klatsch: Zur Sozialform der diskreten Indiskretion*, Berlin and New York: de Gruyter.

Bergmann, J. R. (1988), 'Haustiere als kommunikative Ressourcen', in H.-G. Soeffner (ed.), *Kultur und Alltag* (Sonderband 6 der *Sozialen Welt*), Göttingen: Otto Schwartz.

Bilmes, J. (1985), '"Why that now?" Two kinds of conversational meaning', *Discourse Processes*, 8, 319–55.

Bühler, K. (1934/1965), *Sprachtheorie – Die Darstellungsfunktion der Sprache*, Jena: Gustav Fischer; Stuttgart: Fischer, 1965.
Button, G. (1987), 'Moving out of closings', in G. Button and J. R. E. Lee (eds), *Talk and Social Organisation*, Clevedon: Multilingual Society.
Button, G. and Casey, N. (1984), 'Generating topic: The use of topic initial elicitors', in J. M. Atkinson and J. Heritage (eds), *Structures of Social Action: Studies in conversation analysis*, Cambridge: Cambridge University Press.
Covelli, L. H. and Murray, S. O. (1980), 'Accomplishing topic change', *Anthropological Linguistics*, 22, 382–9.
Craig, R. T. and Tracy, K. (eds) (1983), *Conversational Coherence: Form, structure, and strategy*, Beverly Hills, Ca.: Sage.
Dascal, M. and Katriel, T. (1979), 'Digressions: A study in conversational coherence', in *PTL: A journal for descriptive poetics and theory of literature*, 4, 203–32.
Erickson, F. (1982), 'Money tree, lasagna bush, salt and pepper: Social construction of topical cohesion in a conversation among Italian-Americans', in D. Tannen (ed.), *Analysing Discourse: Text and talk* (GURT, 1981), Washington, DC: Georgetown University Press.
Garfinkel, H. and Sacks, H. (1970), 'On formal structures of practical actions', in J. C. McKinney and E. A. Tiryakian (eds), *Theoretical Sociology. Perspectives and Developments*, New York: Appleton-Century-Crofts.
Goffman, E. (1976), 'Replies and responses', in E. Goffman, *Forms of Talk*, reprinted 1981, Oxford: Blackwell.
Goffman, E. (1979), 'Footing', in E. Goffman, *Forms of Talk*, Oxford: Blackwell, 1981.
Gumperz, J. J., Aulakh, G. and Kaltman, H. (1982), 'Thematic structure and progression in discourse', in J. J. Gumperz (ed.), *Language and Social Identity*, Cambridge: Cambridge University Press.
Heritage, J. C. (1985), 'Recent developments in conversation analysis', *Sociolinguistics*, 15, 1–19.
Heritage, J. C. and Watson, D. R. (1979), 'Formulations as conversational objects', in G. Psathas (ed.), *Everyday Language: Studies in ethnomethodology*, New York: Irvington; New York and Chichester: Wiley.
Heyman, R. D. (1986), 'Formulating topic in the classroom', in *Discourse Processes*, 9, 37–55.
Jefferson, G. (1972), 'Side sequences', in D. Sudnow (ed.), *Studies in Social Interaction*, New York: Free Press; London: Collier-Macmillan.
Jefferson, G. (1984), 'On stepwise transition from talk about a trouble to inappropriately next-positioned matters', in J. M. Atkinson and J. Heritage (eds), *Structures of Social Action: Studies in conversation analysis*, Cambridge: Cambridge University Press.
Keenan, E. O. and Schieffelin, B. B. (1976), 'Topic as a discourse notion: A study of topic in the conversations of children and adults', in C. Li (ed.), *Subject and Topic*, New York: Academic Press.
Luhmann, N. (1975), 'Einfache Sozialsysteme', in N. Luhmann, *Soziologische Aufklärung 2: Aufsätze zur Theorie der Gesellschaft*, Opladen: Westdeutscher Verlag.
Malinowski, B. (1946), 'The problem of meaning in primitive languages', Supplement 1 to C. K. Ogden and I. R. Richards, *The Meaning of Meaning*, 8th edn, London: Kegan Paul, Trench, Trubner and Co., p. 315.

Maynard, D. (1980), 'Placement of topic change in conversation', *Semiotica*, 30, 3/4, 263–90.
Ochs, E. (1979), 'Planned and unplanned discourse', in T. Givón (ed.), *Syntax and Semantics*, vol. 12, *Discourse and Syntax*, New York: Academic Press.
Planalp, S. and Tracy, K. (1980), '"Not to change the topic but . . .": A cognitive approach to the management of conversation', in: D. Nimmo (ed.), *Communication Yearbook 4*, New Brunswick: Transaction Publishers.
Pomerantz, A. (1984), 'Agreeing and disagreeing with assessments: Some features of preferred/dispreferred turn shapes', in J. M. Atkinson and J. Heritage (eds), *Structures of Social Action: Studies in conversation analysis*, Cambridge: Cambridge University Press.
Sacks, H. (1967/68), Unpublished lectures, University of California, Irvine, 1967–8.
Sacks, H., Schegloff, E. and Jefferson, G. (1974), 'A simplest systematics for the organization of turn-taking for conversation', *Language*, 50, 696–735.
Schegloff, E. A. (1971), 'Notes on a conversational practice: Formulating place', in P. P. Giglioli (ed.), *Language and Social Context*, Harmondsworth: Penguin, 1972.
Schegloff, E. A. (1979), 'The relevance of repair to syntax-for-conversation', in T. Givón (ed.), *Syntax and Semantics, vol. 12: Discourse and Syntax*, New York: Academic Press.
Schegloff, E. A. and Sacks, H. (1973), 'Opening up closings', in R. Turner (ed.), *Ethnomethodology*, Harmondsworth: Penguin, 1974.
Schutz, A. (1967), *The Phenomenology of the Social World*, trans. G. Walsh and F. Lehnert (Northwestern University Studies in Phenomenology and Existential Philosophy), Evanston, Ill.: Northwestern University Press.
Schulz, A. and Luckmann, T. (1973/1974), *The Structures of the Life-World*, trans. R. M. Zaner and H. T. Engelhardt jr, 1973, Evanston, Ill.: Northwestern University Press; London: Heinemann, 1974.
Simmel, G. (1908), *Soziologie: Untersuchungen über die Formen der Vergesellschaftung*, Leipzig and Berlin: Duncker and Humblot. Partly trans. into English and ed. by Kurt Wolff, *The Sociology of Georg Simmel*, New York: Free Press; London: Collier-Macmillan, 1950.
Simmel, G. (1917/1950), 'Die Geselligkeit (Beispiel der reinen oder formalen Soziologie)', in G. Simmel, *Grundfragen der Soziologie: Individuum und Gesellschaft*, Leipzig and Berlin: de Gruyter. Partly trans. into English and ed. by Kurt Wolff, *The Sociology of Georg Simmel*, New York: Free Press; London: Collier-Macmillan, 1950.
Tracy, K. (1984), 'Staying on topic: An explication of conversational relevance', *Discourse Processes*, 7, 447–64.
Trevarthen, C. and Hubley, P. (1978), 'Secondary intersubjectivity: Confidence, confiding, and acts of meaning in the first year', in A. Lock (ed.), *Action, Gesture and Symbol: The emergence of language*, London and New York: Academic Press.
West, J. [Withers, C.] (1945), *Plainville, U.S.A.: On life in a rural community of the U.S.A.*, New York: Columbia University Press.
Wilson, J. (1987), 'On the topic of conversation as a speech event', *Research on Language and Social Interaction*, 21, 93–114.
Wylie, L. (1957), *Village in the Vaucluse*, Cambridge, Mass.: Harvard University Press; 2nd edn 1964, 3rd edn 1974.

Name index

Note When a reference is given as, e.g., 164n, please refer to the note(s) to that page at the end of the chapter.

Adamson, L. 45
Adato, A. 210
Adelswärd, V. 161, 162, 164, 164n, 169, 172, 174–5
Agar, M. 168, 172
Als, H. 45
Altorfer, A. 197
Anderson, A. 35, 36, 143
Anna Karénina, 7
Apel, K. O. 114
Argyle, M. 38
Aristotle, 11
Aronsson, K. 161, 162, 169
Atkinson, J. M. 55n, 60
Auer, P. 213n, 223
Aulakh, G. 203n, 222

Baker, G. P. 93
Bakhtin, M. M. 4, 12, 17, 53n, 58, 59, 63, 71–8, 85, 96, 98, 106, 108, 135, 142, 144, 148, 149, 150, 159
Baldwin, D. 168
Baldwin, J. M. 3, 12, 68
Bales, R. F. 159
Bartsch, R. 99, 101
Barwise, J. 14, 86, 87, 93, 96
Bateson, G. 84
Bauman, R. 79
Beach, W. A. 181, 186
Becker, H. S. 33, 40
Bem, D. 36
Beneveniste, E. 51
Berger, P. L. 148, 224
Bergman, Ingmar 100–1
Bergmann, J. R. 53n, 59, 141, 184, 215n, 216n, 218n, 224
Billig, M. 122
Bilmes, J. 214
Birdwhistell, R. L. 6
Blonski, P. P. 64
Blumenthal, A. L. 28
Boas, F. 29
Bourdieu, P. 78–9
Bråten, S. 95–6
Brazelton, T. B. 140
Bruner, J. S. 45, 46n, 59, 162
Bühler, K. 111–13, 123, 205
Button, G. 223
Buttrick, S. 99

Cameron, D. 106
Čapek, K. 4, 10
Caplow, T. 25
Cartwright, D. 25
Casey, N. 211n, 223
Chomsky, N. 12, 28, 31

Name index

Cicourel, A. 148
Clark, H. H. 99, 100, 113, 179
Clark, K. 72, 74
Condillac, E. B. de 12
Converse, P. E. 37
Cook, M. 38
Cooley, C. H. 51n, 59
Costall, A. 12
Coulthard, R. M. 106, 130
Count, E. W. 49n, 59
Covelli, L. H. 204
Craig, R. T. 188–9, 203
Cranach, M. von 179, 181
Crow, B. K. 180–1

Danes, F. 114
Danet, B. 164
Darwin, D. 8, 27, 28, 40
Dascal, M. 203n, 222
Davis, K. E. 15, 42
Davydov, V. V. 13–14
Descartes, 11, 28, 30, 31, 94
Deutsch, M. 170
Dewey, J. 2, 34
Dore, J. 46
Dostoevsky, F. 85
Drew, P. 130, 164
Dreyfus, H. L. 86
Dunstan, R. 164
Durkheim, E. 39, 41

Edmonsen, C. 106
Emerson, C. 72, 74, 75, 77
Erickson, F. 213n, 223
Eroms, H. W. 114

Fanshel, D. 130
Farr, R. M. 8, 9, 15, 16, 26, 29, 32, 33, 35, 36, 38, 39, 143
Farrell, T. B. 196–7
Fichte, J. G. 132
Fillmore, C. J. 149
Flores, C. F. 12, 86
Foppa, K. 9, 14, 19, 99, 141, 178, 179, 180, 181, 185, 203
Forgas, J. 170
Frege, G. 93, 94
Friedman, N. 30

Gadamer, H. G. 85, 88, 152
Gallie, W. B. 31

Garfinkel, H. 204n, 222
Garrod, S. C. 36
Geer, B. 33, 40
Gibson, J. J. 132
Goffmann, E. 15, 34, 36, 40, 41, 54, 203n, 215, 222
Gordan, V. M. 65
Graumann, C. F. 2, 6, 8, 17, 97, 107–8, 109, 110, 111, 113, 117, 120, 167, 190
Greatbatch, D. L. 164n, 173, 174
Grice, H. P. 108, 121
Gugler, B. 179
Gumperz, J. J. 82, 186–7, 203n, 222
Gurwitsch, A. 109
Gustavsson, L. 99, 136, 140, 157, 158, 161, 164, 167, 172

Hacker, F. 93
Halisch, F. 179
Halliday, M. A. K. 54
Harris, E. E. 132
Hegel, G. W. F. 3, 14, 29, 30, 31, 88, 132
Heider, F. 15, 37–9
Heisenberg, W. 91, 92
Henne, H. 106
Heraclitus, 11
Herbst, D. 88–9, 92, 132
Herder, J. G. 2, 4, 11, 29
Heritage, J. 130, 148, 150, 152, 159, 160, 162, 164n, 173, 174, 178, 203n, 204n, 222
Herrmann, T. 106, 107, 108
Heyman, R. D. 204n, 222
Hobbs, J. R. 168
Hockett, C. F. 46n, 59
Holquist, M. 3, 72, 74, 75, 76, 77
Hopper, R. 152
Hubley, P. 46, 46n, 59, 205n, 223
Humboldt, W. von 4, 5, 7, 9, 29, 53n, 59, 133
Husserl, E. 97, 109
Hutchins, E. 67

Ichheiser, G. 15, 36, 39, 41, 111
Indermühle, K. 179
Irvine, J. T. 79
Iser, W. 53n, 59

Jacques, F. 107

Name index

Jakobson, R. 135
James, W. 180
Jauss, H. R. 53n, 59
Jefferson, G. 54, 130, 131, 203n, 206n, 209n, 211n, 213n, 222, 223
Johnson-Laird, P. N. 93
Jolly, A. 46n, 59
Jones, E. E. 15, 33, 35, 42
Jönsson, L. 159–60, 160–1
Juvonen, P. 136, 140, 157, 158, 161, 164, 172

Kalbermatten, U. 179
Kaltman, H. 203n, 222
Kaplan, S. J. 170
Karcevskij, S. 6, 134, 135
Käsermann, M. L. 178, 179, 181, 197
Katriel, T. 203n, 222
Keenan, E. O. 203n, 205, 222
Kellner, H. 216n, 224
Klein, W. 98, 100
Kleist, H. von 190
Köhler, I. 29, 65
Koslowski, B. 140
Kozulin, A. 86
Kreckel, M. 130
Kripke, S. 99
Kuhl, J. 179
Kuhn, T. S. 143

Labov, W. 130
Laing, R. D. 111
Lampi, M. 170n, 172
Lazarus, M. 8
Lee, A. R. 111
Levelt, W. J. M. 106
Levinson, S. C. 130
Lewin, K. 37, 110
Lewontin, R. C. 13
Lieberman, P. 46n, 59
Linell, P. 11, 12, 18–19, 56n, 57n, 60, 67, 94, 99, 102, 137, 140, 143, 150, 156–7, 158, 160–1, 162, 163–4, 163–4n, 172, 174, 190, 192–4
Linneweber, V. 117
Litt, T. 17–18, 110–11
Logotheti, K. 96
Löschper, G. 117

Luckmann, T. 3, 6, 16, 18, 28, 29, 46, 46n, 48n, 51, 52n, 59n, 59, 60, 67, 93, 96, 111, 140, 148, 150n, 157–8, 172, 173, 174, 179, 205, 207
Luhmann, N. 211n, 223
Luria, A. R. 62, 65, 66, 70
Lyons, J. 112

Main, M. 140
Malinowski, B. 215
Mannheim, K. 39, 114
Markovà, I. 6, 11, 12, 14, 18, 25, 28, 29, 30, 32, 38, 63, 71, 74, 83–4, 88, 99, 131, 132, 140, 148, 149, 151, 178
Markus, H. 122–3
Marx, K. 64
Maturana, H. P. 95, 152–3
Maynard, D. 211n, 223
Mead, G. H. 2, 5–6, 8, 12, 15, 16, 17–18, 26–8, 29, 31, 32, 34–5, 35, 36–7, 38, 40, 41, 45, 50–1, 59, 84–5, 110, 135, 138, 178
Mecacci, L. 62
Mehrabian, A. 120
Menzel, H. 86
Meyer, M. F. 30, 38
Middleton, D. 67
Minick, N. 68, 79
Mishler, E. G. 167
Moesch, K. 185, 186
Morawetz, A. 194–6
Morris, C. W. 26, 27
Moscovici, S. 39
Mühlemann, T. 185
Mukařovský, J. 3, 4, 6, 10, 19, 135, 137, 141
Mummendey, A. 117
Murray, S. O. 204

Naess, A. 84
Newcomb, T. W. 37
Nietzsche, F. 76, 117
Nisbett, R. E. 15, 33, 35, 42

Ochs, E. 79, 219
Osgood, C. E. 107
Ostrom, T. M. 111
Otten, S. 117

Peirce, C. S. 31
Perry, J. 14, 86, 96
Philips, S. 79
Phillipson, H. 111
Piaget, J. 10, 45, 68
Pied Piper, 16–17, 141
Pike, K. 106
Planalp, S. 203n, 222
Plato, 11, 111–12
Pomerantz, A. M. 130, 160, 213n, 223
Putnam, H. 95

Radzikhovskii, L. A. 63–4
Raskolnikov, 85
Rasmussen, P. 88, 92
Reddy, M. 149–50
Rehbock, H. 106
Rogoff, B. 67
Rommetveit, R. 4, 6, 12–13, 14, 17, 28, 32, 59n, 60, 83, 86, 91, 93, 94, 98, 100, 113, 114, 131, 132, 135, 148, 149–50, 152, 156, 173, 190
Rorty, R. 83–4, 164
Ross, L. 42
Rousseau, J. J. 12
Rundström, B. 162
Russell, B. 14

Sacks, H. 54, 130, 203, 204n, 206, 206n, 209n, 210–11n, 213, 222, 223
Sakharov, L. S. 70
Sapir, E. 29
Sätterlund-Larsson, U. 160–1
Saussure, F. 134
Schaefer, E. F. 99, 113, 179
Schaffer, H. R. 140
Schegloff, E. A. 54, 130, 152, 163, 172, 180, 203n, 203, 209n, 213, 222
Schieffelin, B. B. 203n, 205, 222
Schilcher, F. von 13
Schutz, A. 2–6, 18, 52–3, 89, 111, 148, 207, 215
Searle, J. R. 90, 96, 129–30, 161, 180
Sebeok, T. A. 107
Sefi, S. 160
Shotter, J. 100

Shreuder, R. 99
Simmel, G. 25, 214–15, 218
Sinclair, J. M. 130
Skinner, B. F. 31–2
Smirnov, A. N. 65
Smirnov, S. D. 64
Sommer, C. M. 115n, 123
Spencer-Brown, L. 14, 87–8, 132
Spinoza, 84
Stebbing, S. 14
Still, A. 12
Stone, C. A. 67
Stutterheim, C. von 98, 100
Süssmilch, J. P. 12

Tarde, J. B. 15
Taylor, T. J. 106
Tennant, N. 13
Todorov, T. 150
Tolstoy, L. 7, 21
Tracy, K. 187–9, 203n, 222
Trevarthen, C. 45–6, 46n, 59, 96, 205n, 222
Tronick, E. 45
Turner, R. H. 37
Tur-Sinai, N. H. 51
Tynjanov, J. 134–5

Uhlenbeck, E. M. 12
Upshaw, H. S. 111

van Peursen, C. A. 110
Varela, F. J. 95, 152–3
Vološinov, V. N. 3, 4, 5, 6, 12, 53n, 59, 71, 74, 85, 96, 135, 136, 149–50
Vossler, C. 76
Vygotsky, L. S. 3, 6, 7, 10, 16–17, 45, 63–71, 77, 78, 79, 85, 86

Walker, G. 194–6
Watson, D. R. 162, 204n, 222
Watson, J. B. 35
Werner, H. 68
Wertsch, J. V. 6, 16, 29, 63, 64, 67, 68, 69, 79, 86, 98, 102, 108, 134n, 135, 144
West, J. 216
Wiemann, J. M. 130
Wiener, M. 120
Wilkes-Gibbs, D. 113

Wilson, J. 210–11n, 223
Winograd, T. 12, 86
Wintermantel, M. 120
Wish, M. 170
Wittgenstein, L. 83, 93
Wold, A. H. 60
Wrong, D. 153
Wunderlich, D. 186–7
Wundt, W. 8, 15, 26–9, 32, 34, 36, 109

Wylie, L. 216n, 224

Yakubinsky, L. P. 7, 9, 10, 85
Youniss, J. 63

Zajonc, R. B. 122–3
Zander, A. 25
Zavalloni, M. 120
Zinchenko, V. P. 64, 65

Subject index

abstraction, 16, 47, 48, 51, 205, 211
actor and observer, 33, 34, 35, 40, 41
analytic units, 187–8, 189, 190
   conceptual and epistemological, 131, 137, 138, 142
   physical, 131, 138, 142
   segmentation into, 185
asymmetric dualism, 134
asymmetry, 147, 155, 157, 160, 172-3
   in dialogue, 172
   global, 158
   interactional, 160, 167, 171
   local, 158
   in roles of speaker and listener, 156
asymmetry/symmetry, 56, 147, 148, 156, 168–70
autopoietic models (systems), 95, 96, 153

behaviour, 32, 38
   contingent (unintentional), 49–50, 54
   interpretation of, 54
behaviourism, 30, 33, 34
   social, 32
   versus mentalism, 30

Cartesian paradigm, 12, 17, 25, 26–7, 28, 29, 30, 31, 32, 38

Cartesian dualism, 26–7, 28, 31
co-genetic logic, 14, 17, 87–8, 89, 90, 94, 95, 132
cognition, 12, 89
   dialogical character of, 122
   multiperspectivity of, 122–3
   social, 122–3
cognitive science, 16, 46, 86, 95
   Cartesian, 32
   criticism of, 16, 83–4, 86, 95
   presuppositions of, 17, 32
communication
   development of, 51
   social, 3, 4, 16, 45, 46, 47, 48–52, 56, 63
communicative acts, 37, 48, 55, 149
   as context-dependent and context-renewing, 149, 150
communicative action, 54, 148, 168
   chains of, 16, 49
   kept alive by disagreements, 214
communicative cultures, 55
communicative genres, 55, 59, 59n, 60
communicative processes
   non-linguistic, 55
   in non-Western cultures, 55
confrontational interaction, 168, 170, 171, 173, 197, 214
consciousness, 85, 86
   social origin, 66, 85
   streams of, 52–3, 56, 58, 215

synchronization of, 52–3, 56, 215
context dependence, 135, 148–9
context sensitivity, 206
convergence of perspectives, 35–6
conversation, 7, 8, 16, 19, 31, 58–9, 130, 131, 135, 137, 171, 172–3, 182, 183, 184, 196
  aimless, 191
  closure of, 211, 213
  context shaped and context renewing, 149, 150
  definition of, 57–8
  degeneration into quarrels, 214
  informal, 184
  initiation of, 213
  as more than the transmission of information, 7
  not bound by formal restrictions, 211
  ordinary, 172–3
  social organization of, 210–11
  as a sub-species of dialogue, 16, 58, 173
  versus dialogue, 58–9
conversation analysis, 36, 54, 130, 150, 173
conversation of gestures, 5, 27–8, 28–9, 45, 138
conversational discontinuity, 211, 213, 216
conversational implicatures, 121–2
co-operation/confrontation, 168, 173, 197

decontextualization, 69, 70, 77, 90, 102, 167
development
  co-development, 131, 140
  cultural, 66, 67, 69, 76
  of language, 57
  socio-historical, 16, 47, 50, 65
  symmetrical and asymmetrical co-development, 140
  topic, 183–4, 201
  triadic, 131
dialegesthai, 106, 116, 121
dialogical
  approach, 83, 86, 87
  closure, 95–6
  interdependence, 131, 149
  meaning, definition, 3–4, 5, 6–7, 9, 55–7, 58

paradigm, 84, 87, 89
perspective, 17, 105
dialogicality, 71, 73, 74, 76, 78, 79, 150–1
  ontogenesis of, 95
dialogism (epistemology), 3, 4–5, 11–12, 14, 20, 63, 74, 131
dialogue, 16, 31, 63, 67, 105–8, 113, 115, 129, 150, 174
  adjacency pairs as units of analysis of, 131
  asymmetry in, 18, 147–8
  as a collective product, 155–6
  conceptualization of partners in, 107–8
  co-verbal aspects of, 182
  definition of, 3–4, 56, 173
  dramatic, 141
  dynamics of the self-organizing principle of, 157–8
  as face-to-face interaction, 1, 4, 6–7, 9, 10, 52, 56, 73, 136
  genetic aspects of, 52, 172
  intentional aspects of, 179
  monologic, 184
  ontogenetic aspects of, 46
  origins of, 46
  physical sub-division of, 131, 137–8
  power and dynamics of, 150
  prior to monologue, 25
  reproductive power of, 152–3
  social construction of, 148
  as socially constructed, 148–9
  structure of, 183
  units of analysis of, 14, 15, 18, 129–31
  universal attributes of, 55–7, 58
  universal form of human communication, 56
  versus conversation, 58–9
  versus monologue, 9, 19
discourse
  analysis, 106, 107
  conversational (gossip), 215–6
  triple intentionality of, 111–12, 113
  unfolding of, 116
divergence of perspectives, 33, 34–5, 36, 40, 112–13, 117, 166
dominance, 157–9, 163–4, 172
  as amount of talk, 158

234 Subject index

dominance – *contd.*
  in conversation and dialogue, 57, 153–7, 163
  dimensions of, 157–8
  interactional, 18, 136, 140, 158–63, 164, 169
  local and global properties in dialogue, 157
  and power relationships, 140
  professional, 161–2
  quantification of, 171
  semantic, 158, 163
  strategic, 158
dyadic character of words or utterances, 136
dynamics of dialogue, 10, 15, 19, 20, 35, 40, 114, 116, 118–9, 121, 140, 149, 178, 179, 181, 196, 197
  analysis of, 15
  monological aspects of, 184, 186
  perspectivity of, 110, 117, 118–19

egocentric speech, 70, 77, 86
embeddedness
  of human cognition, 86
  of mind, 84–5, 95, 96, 102
  situational, 52, 207
  of two kinds of speech, 136, 140
  of utterances, 130, 131, 151
emotional state, 197
environment
  local, 202, 206, 207
  sequential, 213
epistemic responsibility, 98, 99
equality and inequality in dialogue, 56–7
ethnomethodology, 1, 150, 151, 157, 172
expression *versus* impression, 40
external relations, 14, 132

face-to-face communication, 1, 4, 6–7, 9, 10, 28, 50, 52–3, 54, 56, 136, 144
fixation of perspectives, 12–3, 17, 92–4, 101
folk psychology
  (*Völkerpsychologie*) 8, 26, 27, 29, 109

genetic
  approach, 78
  domains, 64–6
  method, 16, 64–5, 68, 78
Gestalt psychology, 36, 88
German expressivism, 1, 2–3, 4, 7, 29
gestures, 8
  conversation of, 5, 27–8, 28–9, 45, 138
  role of in development of language, 8
  role of in development of self, 26
  synchronization of, 140
gossip, 215–6

hearer's commitment, 166, 169
Hegelian paradigm, 25, 29, 30, 31, 32, 38, 88, 149
hermeneutic methods, 83
horizon, 109, 110
  inner and outer, 109
  of meaning, 121

illocutionary acts, 180
immediacy, 52, 53, 56
impression *versus* expression, 40, 41
impressions, 39, 40, 41
individual and environment, 132–3
  co-development of, 132–3
  interdependence of, 2, 132–3
individualism, 6, 12, 69
  psychological, 107
information-processing models/ paradigm, 7, 8, 40, 106, 107
  as basically monological, 106, 122
initiative and response (IR) 18–9, 99, 136–7, 138, 143, 147, 149, 151–2, 153, 155, 157, 158, 164
  interplay of, 150
  IR analysis, 18–9, 158, 164
  IR difference, 159
  IR measures, 174
instinct, 49, 55
institutional contexts, 163, 164, 169, 173
institutional interactions, 169, 173, 216–7
institutionalized procedures and rules, 157, 161–2, 164–5, 216

Subject index

intentional states, 180
intentions, 19, 112, 179, 180
　communicative, 49, 179, 183
　conceptual problems, 19
　identification of in dialogues, 179–80
　interactive, 178, 182, 191–2, 196
　role in communication, 19
　specific intentions, absence of, 183–4, 195, 197, 198
　strategic, 19, 182, 184, 191, 194, 195, 197
　'what' intentions, 180, 181, 185, 188
　'what for' intentions, 180, 181, 182, 183, 188, 189–90, 196, 198
intentionality, 16, 47, 51–2, 112
　triple nature of in dialogue, 111–12, 113
interactional dominance, 18, 136, 143, 157, 158
interdependence
　dialogical, 131, 149
　of individual and environment, 2, 88, 132–3
internal relations, 14, 18, 132, 135, 136, 139
internal representation models, 93, 95
internalization, 16–7
　of speech, 10
interpsychological plane of cultural development, 16–7, 66–7, 68, 71, 77–8
intersubjectivity, 51, 53, 97, 113, 137, 148
　'origo' of, 113
intersubjective mirroring, 51n, 59, 96
intrapsychological plane of cultural development, 16–17, 66–7, 68, 71, 77–8

Janus-like nature of utterances, 137, 150–1, 154
joint-attention, 113

language, 31, 45, 72, 74–5, 90–1, 129
　appropriation of, 75, 135

　as both permanent and transient, 134
　Cartesian assumptions of, 48
　as the central system of social communication, 49
　collective and individual poles of, 134, 135
　dialogical conception of, 135
　national, 74–5
　ordinary, 90, 94, 98
　origins in gestures, 27–8
　social, 77–8, 78–9
　as a social phenomenon, 29, 135
　as a system of signs, 45
　as a tool or instrument, 112
　written bias of, 94
learning, institutionalized, 63, 78–9
Lebenswelt (life-world), 92, 99, 101, 111
linguistic code, 49
　genetic transmission of, 49
　the result of social interaction, 49
local
　context, 206
　environment, 202, 206, 207
　reciprocity, 156
local sensitivity, 19, 184
　concept of, 206–7
　control of, 215–17
　as organizing conversation, 210–11
　principle of, 205–6
logic
　Boolean, 93
　co-genetic, 14, 17, 18, 87–8, 89, 90, 93, 94, 95, 132
　dialectic, 14, 132
　dialogical, 14, 132
　of external relations, 14
　formal, 131
　Hegelian, 14, 88
　of internal relations, 14, 132–3

meaning
　co-determination of, 3, 135, 136
　common core of, 53
　as context dependent, 148–9
　as culturally inherited, 148
　implicit, 122
　joint construction of, 136
　'literal', 93–4

Subject index

mediation, semiotic, 68–9, 71, 79
mediational means, 69, 77
microgenesis, 65
mind, 2, 28–9, 32, 45, 95
   and behaviour, 32–3, 38
   dialogical origin of, 84
   dialogicality of, 95
   social model of, 26, 27
   socio-cultural approach to, 17, 62–3, 65–6, 71, 72, 78, 79
monological
   approach, 83
   models, 83, 106
   situation, 189
monologism, 5, 9, 11, 17
monologue
   meaning of term, nature of, 5, 6, 9
   as really dialogue, 9, 137
   versus dialogue, 9, 19
moves
   controlling, 159, 161, 163
   directing, 159
   inhibiting, 159, 161, 163
multivoicedness (heteroglossia), 75–6, 142, 143

neutral local coherence, 141, 188–9, 190, 191, 192, 193, 195, 196, 197, 198

ontogenesis, 65, 66, 69
   of dialogicity, 95

perspective, 98, 99, 101, 140
   of actor, 36, 38
   co-determination of, 135
   co-development of, 140
   communication of, 114
   convergence of, 35, 36
   dialogical, 105, 112
   divergence of, 33, 34, 35, 36, 40, 112–13, 117, 166
   dominance of actor or observer, 34–5
   dynamics of, 110, 116–17
   evolution of, 113–14
   fixation of, 12–13, 17, 92–4, 101
   giving and taking, interplay of, 111, 114
   individual and common, 135
   national values in, 117–20
   of observer, 34
   personal values in, 117–20
   phenomenological explication, 109
   reciprocity of, 110–11
   relativity of, 13, 87, 88, 89, 90–2, 95, 101
   setting of, 18, 97, 121, 164–5, 167
   structure of, 109
   taking, 2–3, 17, 18, 110, 114, 135, 167
   terminology of, 108–9
   understanding by pupil or layperson, 166–7
perspectivity, 20, 193
   dynamics of, 110
   omnipresence of, 17
phatic communion, 215
phenomenology, 1, 109
phenomenological approaches, 2, 109
phylogenesis, 52, 65
power, 56, 152–3
   and dynamics of dialogue, 150
   social, 52, 153, 163, 174
Prague School of linguistics, 114
Prague School of semiotics, 134, 135
propositional acts, 180
proto-signs, 51–2

quarrels, 170, 171, 214

rationalism *versus* empiricism, 30–1
recipient design, 54
reciprocity, 16, 46, 47, 48, 50, 51, 52–3, 56, 140
   of perspectives, 2, 110–11
   prelinguistic, 46, 46n, 59
relations
   external, 14, 132
   internal, 14, 18, 132, 133, 135, 136, 139
repair actions, 54
repairs
   other-, 180
   self-, 180
representational models, 86
responsibility, 147
   epistemic, 98, 99
   professional, 167–8

speaker's and recipient's, 155–6, 166, 169
  in social encounters, 167
ritual, function of, 218–9
role
  of hearer and speaker, 107, 108, 115, 156
  taking, 110
'role' concept of dialogue partners, 107–8
routinized activity, 50, 55

self, 31, 84, 111
  development of, 8, 26–7, 38
  emergence of, 26
  as object, 26
  and other, 30, 31, 37–8
  presentation of, 41
  regulation of, 41
  social origin, 173
self–other duality, 30, 96
self-perception, 37, 38
self-repairs, 180
semantics
  formal, 86
  truth-conditional, 89, 90–1, 92
semantic dominance, 158, 163
semantic reversals, 141–2, 143
semiotic mediation, 63, 68–9, 71, 79
semioticians, 6, 12, 16, 64
semiotics, 150
signs, 52, 67, 68, 113, 123, 134
  mediation by, 67
  proto-, 51-2
  psychological tools, 68
  system of, 1, 45, 50
situative context, 202, 205
social
  interaction, 1, 4, 37, 39, 40–1, 52
  language, 75, 77–8, 78–9
  power, 52, 153, 163
  realities temporarily shared, 98, 102
social communication, 3, 4, 16, 45, 46, 47, 48–52, 56, 63
  evolution of, 48–9
  genetic aspects, 5, 45
  natural *versus* historic, 48–9
social construction
  of communication, 50
  of dialogue, 149

sociality, 16, 47, 48, 74, 214
socio-cultural approach to mind, 17, 62–3, 65–6, 71, 72, 78, 79
speakers and hearers, 73, 107–8
speaker's responsibility and recipient's commitment, 166, 169
speech
  as action, 15
  dialogical quality of, 141
  embeddedness, two kinds of, 136
  inner (egocentric), 70, 77, 86
  internalization of, 10
  as reflexion of mind, 15
speech acts, triple intention of, 111–12
speech act theory, 129
speech genres, 76, 78, 79
strategic goals, 183, 184, 189
symbolic interaction(ism), 1, 18, 28, 84
symbolic nature of human communication, 3, 4, 5
symmetry/asymmetry, 56, 147, 148, 156, 168–70

tertium comparationis, 134
three-step processes, 130–2, 133, 134, 135
  different levels of, 136, 143
three-step units
  analysis of, 99, 138–40
  analysis across turns, 141, 143
  as turns, 136–8
topic, 98, 99–100, 101, 115, 201, 202, 203
  change of, 141, 207–10
  and comment, 112–13
  constraints, 203–4
  differentiation of, 99
  evolution of perspective of, 113
  expansion of, 187
  formulation of, 204, 205
  joint production of, 204, 205
  maintenance of, 19, 203, 205
  management of, 187, 190, 191, 205
  monological aspects of, 184, 186
  progression, 19, 183, 184, 188, 189, 190, 198, 203, 205

topic – *contd.*
  turn-internal processes in, 184, 186, 188–90
topicalization of local matters, 19, 205, 207, 210, 213
translinguistics, 72–3, 74
'trigger' topics, 213, 214
turns, 129, 130, 131, 136, 141, 173
  analysis across, 141
  retroactive and proactive parts of, 137
  as three-step units, 136–8
turn-internal processes, 141, 187, 188, 189, 190
turn sequences, 129, 140
turn-taking, 19, 130, 172, 182, 203

universal attributes of dialogue, 55–7, 58
utterance, 72, 73, 76–7, 114, 129, 130, 149, 150, 157
  as belonging both to a voice and to others, 73
  dyadic features of, 136
  embeddedness of, 151
  inherently dialogical, 72
  Janus-like nature of, 137, 150–1, 154, 156
  meaning of, 73
  the real unit of speech communication, 72
  retroactive and proactive, 136, 137
  as unit, 72, 73, 106, 129
utterance-understanding-context triad, 149

verb as analytic unit, 185
ventriloquation, 75, 77, 78
voice, 17, 72, 74, 76, 77, 85, 98, 108, 113, 122
voicedness, multi- (heteroglossia), 75–6, 142, 143
Völkerpsychologie (folk psychology), 8, 26, 27, 29, 109
word
  as two-sided acts, 135, 136
  appropriation of, 135